ISBN 978-1-0694303-1-1
Edited by Inayah Masood
Cover design by Essa Masood
Created by Dr. Humaira Mehboob

Acknowledgments

The completion of this compilation would not have been possible without the support, guidance, and encouragement of many individuals.

I would like to express my sincere gratitude to my mentor, Dr. Afsheen Mehar, who originally coined the term '2-minute drill' and whose instruction and insight laid the foundation for much of the content included in this collection.

I also wish to acknowledge Dr. Sarah Tahir, whose collaboration, discussions, and shared resources greatly enriched my learning experience and contributed meaningfully to the development of these notes.

Special thanks are extended to Dr. Asmara Khan, whose careful review and thoughtful suggestions helped refine the structure of this material.

I am deeply grateful to my editor, Inayah Masood, for her careful attention to detail, constructive feedback, and endless patience throughout the process of preparing this work. Her support has been invaluable in helping shape this collection into its final form.

Finally, I am deeply thankful to my family for their unwavering support and encouragement throughout this process.

This collection is the result of collective effort, shared knowledge, and way too many highlighters.

for my father.

Table of Contents

Obstetrics/ Gynecology **8**

Primary Amenorrhea 15

Secondary Amenorrhea 19

Vaginal Bleeding 21

Vaginal Bleeding in First Trimester (T1-T2) 23

Vaginal Bleeding in Third Trimester (T3) 25

Vaginal Bleeding - Elderly 26

Polycystic Ovarian Syndrome (POS) 27

Pelvic Pain 28

Infertility 29

Hirsutism 31

Vaginal Discharge 32

Preeclampsia 33

Abortion 34

Menopause 35

Osteoporosis 36

Cardiovascular/ Respiratory System **38**

Chest Pain 43

Chest Pain - Myocardial Infarction 45

Chest Pain - Aortic Dissection 46

Chest Pain - Pericarditis 47

Chest Pain - GERD 48

Chest Pain - Aortic Stenosis 50

Chest Pain - Pulmonary Embolism 51

Chest Pain - Pneumothorax 53

Heart Racing 54

Atrial Fibrillation (AF) 56

Hypertension 58

Syncope 60

Congestive Heart Failure (CHF) 62

Deep Vein Thrombosis (DVT) 63

Peripheral Artery Disease (PAD) 65

Cough 67

Hemoptysis 68

Asthma 70
COPD 72
Pediatrics 74
Cough 80
Vomiting 81
Diarrhea - Acute 82
Diarrhea - Chronic 83
Diarrhea - Bloody 84
Constipation 86
Enuresis 88
Hematuria 90
Jaundice 92
Crying Baby 94
Failure to Thrive 96
Delayed Speech 98
Autism 100
Attention Deficit Hyperactivity Disorder (ADHD) 101
Anemia 104
Sudden Infant Death Syndrome (SIDS) 105
Allergy/Anaphylaxis 106
Nephrotic Syndrome 107
Hyperreactive airway Disease 109
Fracture 111
Sleep Disorder 113
Rash 116
Febrile Seizure 118
Obesity 120
Musculoskeletal System 121
Single Joint Pain 127
Multiple Joint Pain 129
Rheumatoid Arthritis 131
Gout 132
Neck Pain 133
Shoulder Pain 135
Carpal Tunnel Syndrome 137

Hip Pain 138
Knee Pain 140
Acute Back Pain 143
Chronic Back Pain 145
Ankle Pain 148
Fatigue 150
Gastrointestinal System 152
Hematemesis/ Melena 157
Acute Diarrhea 159
Chronic Diarrhea 160
Bloody Diarrhea 162
Acute Abdominal Pain 164
Abdominal Pain — Elderly 166
Chronic Abdominal Pain 167
Bright Red Blood Per rectum (BRBPR) 169
Dysphagia 171
Jaundice 174
Urinary System 176
Hematuria 181
Urinary incontinence 183
Stress Incontinence 185
Erectile Dysfunction 186
Penile Discharge 188
Benign Prostatic Hyperplasia (BPH) 189
Lower UTI 190
Renal Colic 192
Lymphadenopathy 194
Scrotal Mass 196
Neurology 198
Headache 203
Tremors 206
Parkinson's Disease 208
Dizziness/Vertigo 209
Gait 211
Concussions 213

Seizures 214
Stroke 216
Subarachnoid Hemorrhage 217
Sleep Apnea 218
Facial Palsy 220
Hoarseness 222
Multiple Sclerosis 224
Psychiatry 225
Panic Attack 231
Depression 232
OCD 233
Mania 235
Schizophrenia 236
Anorexia Nervosa 237
Dementia 239
Delirium 241
Suicide 243
Insomnia 244
Fatigue 245

Obstetrics/ Gynecology

How to organise yourself before entering the station + Key 10

Primary Amenorrhea 16

Secondary Amenorrhea 20

Vaginal Bleeding 22

Vaginal Bleeding in First Trimester (T1-T2) 24

Vaginal Bleeding in Third Trimester (T3). 26

Vaginal Bleeding - Elderly 27

Polycystic Ovarian Syndrome (POS) 28

Pelvic Pain. 29

Infertility 30

Hirsutism 32

Vaginal Discharge 33

Preeclampsia 34

Abortion. 35

Menopause 36

Osteoporosis. 37

How to organise yourself before entering the station

Before entering the station, you will have under two minutes to read the prompt and jot down notes in your booklet.

These notes should focus on key information you'll need to remember while taking the history from the standardized participant (SP). The SP is an actor trained to portray a specific medical condition or scenario. Their purpose is to interact with you and allow the physician examiner (PE) to observe and assess your performance.

The booklet provided is rectangular, about half the size of an A4 sheet. It contains blank sheets for your notes, as well as candidate code stickers, which you'll need to hand over to the examiner before starting each station.

Given the time constraints and anxiety during the station, these notes can serve as a valuable guide to help you complete a thorough history.

Therefore, it is essential to practice responding to prompts and mastering the '2-minute drill' regularly to achieve your best results.

HOW TO PRACTICE :

For practice purposes, folding an A4 sheet in half works well to simulate the booklet.

Hence this book is divided into two columns:

Left column	Right column
Contains a breakdown of the mnemonics and the questions you may need to ask.	Notes to write in your booklet as part of your 2-minute drill, often including mnemonics that make the best use of your time and help you recall essential steps efficiently!

These structured notes will provide a clear and concise roadmap to ensure you stay focused and efficient during the station.

The KEY

Knock on the door, Walk in, Wear a smile, Greet the examiner, and hand the candidate code, *"Hi, here's my candidate code."*
Sanitize your hands and simultaneously:

Introduce yourself to the standardized participant (SP):
"Hello, I am Dr___ and I will be your physician today. May I know your name and age, please? How would you like to be addressed? That's great!

"Is it okay if I sit down and take a few notes?"

PC: Presenting Complaints
"What brings you in here today?"
Listen to the patient. It is important to express **Empathy.**
"I am sorry to hear that. That must be quite distressing."

"Okay, so I would like to ask you a few questions and do a physical exam after and we will figure out a treatment plan for you today!"

SOCRATES-B: For conditions with other symptoms SOCRATES-B can still be used.

- site: *"Where is the pain? Can you point at it?"*
- onset: *"Was it gradual or sudden in onset?"*
- character: *"What kind of pain is it? Is it a dull pain or a sharp pain?"*
- radiate: *"Does the pain radiate anywhere?"*
- associated symptoms: *"Any associated symptoms?"*
- time: *"Is the pain constant or intermittent?"*
- exacerbating factor: *"Does anything relieve the pain or make it worse?"*
- severity: *"On a scale from 1-10, how would you rate the pain? 10 being the worst."*
- before: *"Have you had this before?"*

Not every P/C involves pain. Some complaints may just require 'o-ate' onset associated s/s, time, and exacerbating/ relieving factors.

COCA-b: For any vomiting/discharge/sputum/stool/urine.
Colour, **O**dor, **Consistency**, **A**mount, **B**lood (If yes for blood, ask **BBL**)

BBL — (if pt complains of bleeding), stands for:

- Blood thinners – *"Are you on blood thinners?"*
- Bloody Diarrhea – *"Do you bruise easily or bleed easily?"*
- Liver Disease — *"Any hx of liver disease?"*

Impact: *"How are you coping with this?"*

DDX: Differentials for the condition given for each condition.

SIGNPOST: This symbol means you have to signpost! A signpost is an introductory statement. This is to introduce your segment of questions, so the examiner is aware of your line of questioning.

E.g.: DDx - means you have to place an introductory statement before asking for differentials: *"I am going to ask a few questions to rule out any other causes."*

Red flags: This is for conditions we need to rule out right away as they may require urgent attention.

PAM HUGS FOSS: stands for:

- Past medical hx: *"Since this is the first time we are meeting; do you have any past medical conditions that I should know about? Or that you have been treated for?"*
- Allergies: *"Do you have any allergies?"*
- Medications: *"Are you on any medications? What are the medications? Are you adherent to your medications? What is the dosage?"*
- Hospitalization/Surgery: *"Have you ever had any hospitalization before? Any surgeries done before?"*
- Urinary changes: *"Have you noticed changes in your urine?"*
- GIT changes: *"Have you noticed any changes in your bowel habits?"*
- SAD- **S**moking/**A**lcohol/Recreational **D**rugs:
    - *"Do you smoke? How many cigarettes a day? For how long? Have you ever thought about quitting?"*
    - *"Do you drink alcohol? How often?"*
    - *"Have you done any recreational drugs? What have you used? How do you take it? Do you sniff or inject? Do you share needles?"*
- Family history: *"Any family history of any medical conditions?"* Specific medical conditions you are concerned about.
- Occupation: *"If I may ask, what do you do for a living?"*
- Social: *"May I know about your living conditions? Who do you live with?"*
- Support: *"Do you have any family around? Are they supportive? That's good to know."*

Mnemonics for system questions:
Obs/Gyne:

MGOS: is for Menstrual, Gynecological, Obstetrics, and Sexual development hx.

Menstrual hx- ACRAL PPPL- stands for:
Age of menarche — *"How old were you when you got your first period?"*
Cycle — *"Can you tell me about your cycle?"*
Regular/irregular — *"Is your cycle regular or irregular?"*
Amount of blood/clots — *"How many pads do you use?"*
Length of cycle — *"How many days do you have the period for?"*
Pelvic pain — *"Do you have any pain during your period?"*
PMS – *"Do you have any hx of bloating? Any headaches? Do you notice any mood changes? Any irritability? Notice any depression?"*
Pap smear/gyne **P**rocedures — (If above 21 years old) *"When was your last pap test? Was it normal?"*
LMP — *"When was your last menstrual period? Any chance you might be Pregnant?"*

Gynecological hx - Starts with **confidentiality** — *"I want you to know that everything we talk about today will remain confidential between us unless it concerns your safety, then I am required by law to report it, OK?"* It is very important to be mindful when asking sensitive questions, it's good to ease in. Taking cues from the patient's response. — **RONDS CA-stands for:**

Recent partners — *"Are you in a relationship? Are you sexually active?"*
sexual **O**rientation — *"If I may ask, do you prefer to be with men or women or both?"*
Number of partners — *"Are you in a monogamous relationship?" If not, "How many partners have you had in the past 12 months?"*
Dyspareunia — *"Do you experience any pain or discomfort during intercourse?"*
Safe sexual practices — *"Do you practice safe sex? By that, I mean using condoms/barrier methods?"*
Contraception — *"Do you use contraception? What type of contraception?"*
Abuse — *"I'd like to ask about your partner, are they supportive?* - pause - *Are you happy in your relationship?"* - If the patient has sexual abuse as an agenda, they will not answer these questions positively. Explore further if deemed necessary. *"Do you feel safe in this relationship? Have you ever been forced to do anything sexual that you were not comfortable with?"*

Obstetric hx - **GT PAL stands for:**

"Have you ever conceived before? Any hx of abortions or miscarriages? Number of babies you have delivered? Was it a vaginal delivery? Any complications? Were all your babies full-term? Any congenital abnormalities?"

<u>**S**exual Development</u> - **BHS** stands for :
Breast development — *"At what age did your breasts develop?"*
Hair growth — *"When did you start to notice hair growth in your pubic area or underarms?"*
growth **S**prout — *"When did you get your growth sprout?"*

(*These are sensitive questions. Start with* ***confidentiality*** *if needed.*
Ease into the conversation:
"Are you in a relationship? Are you sexually active? Is it a monogamous relationship? Do you feel any pain during intercourse? Any history of sexually transmitted diseases? Do you use contraceptives? What kind? How long?)

<u>**Menopause Hx**</u> - Ask about the age of menopause. *"When was your last menstrual period?* (Need 12 months of a menstrual-free period to diagnose menopause) —
Vu Fidl BB stands for:
V -Vaginal symptoms — Dryness, bleedings d/c, pruritus, dyspareunia.*"Have you ever experienced any vaginal irritation? Any itchiness? Any dc (*If yes, ask **COCA-B**)
U - Urinary Changes — *"Have you experienced any urinary changes? Any burning during*
F - hot Flashes — *"Have you experienced any hot flashes?"*
I - Insomnia — *"Do you have difficulty falling asleep?"*
D -Depression — *"How has your mood been lately? Have you felt your mood has been low? Have you noticed that you are not interested in things you used to be interested in before?*
L - decreased Libido (ask sexual hx)
B - Bleeding — *"Have you had any spotting or bleeding?"*
B - Bone pain — *"Any hx of bone pain or joint pain? Any f/hx of osteoporosis?"*

COLD NUT (*if suspecting endometrial carcinoma) stands for:*

- <u>C</u> - Hx of Cancer
- <u>O</u> - Obesity: *"What do you say your ideal weight is?"*
- <u>L</u> - Late menopause: *"When was your LMP?"*
- <u>D</u> - DM: *"Have you been diagnosed with DM? Do you feel thirsty a lot? Have you noticed that you pee a lot?"*
- <u>N</u> - Nulliparity: *"Have you ever conceived? Do you have any children?"*
- <u>U</u> - Unopposed Estrogen (PCOs/OCP/HRT)
- <u>T</u> - Tamoxifen: *"Are you on any medication like Tamoxifen? Are you taking any contraceptive pills?"*

BBL – (if pt complains of bleeding), stands for :

- <u>B</u> - Blood thinners – *"Are you on blood thinners?"*
- <u>B</u> - Bloody Diarrhea – *"Do you bruise easily or bleed easily?"*
- <u>L</u> - Liver Disease — *"Any hx of liver disease?"*

PREGNANT FEMALE HISTORY TAKING:

PPF Chun VbL

- P - Planned — *"Was this a planned pregnancy?"*
- P - Partner — *"Is your partner involved?"*
- F - Feeling — *"How do you feel about it?"*
- C - Congratulate, if pt is happy with being pregnant — *"Well, congratulations! I'm happy for you!"*
- H - Health — *"How is your general health?"*
- U - Urinary Changes — *"Any changes in your urine? Eg increased frequency?"*
- N- Nausea — *"Any nausea?"*
- V - Vomiting — *"Any vomiting?"*
- B - Breast Engorgement — *"Any breast engorgement?"*
- L - Last Menstrual Period — *"When was your last menstrual period?"*

ABCDE

- Fetal Activity — *"Do you feel the baby kick?"* (ask in T3)
- Bleeding/ Cramps — *"Have you noticed any bleeding? Any abdominal cramps?*
- Discharge — *"Any vaginal discharge?"* If yes, ask **COCA-b.**
- Expected Due Date — *"When is the expected due date?"*

Antenatal Case →

- *"Have you had regular antenatal checkups?"*
- *"Did you get screened for infections?"*
- *"Have you had your U/S done?"*
- *"Do you know the # babies ?"*
- *"Do you know about the location of the placenta?"*

Primary Amenorrhea

Pt has never had a period

SOCRATES + **MGOS hx**

SIGN POST *"Just to make sure there's nothing serious going on."*

"Secondary sexual characteristics present?" If ***YES***:

imperforate Hymen, AIS, Mullerian Agenesis, Prolactinoma, Thyroid, Pregnancy

H A M P T P

SIGN POST DDx: *"I'd like to ask you a few questions to rule out other causes."*

Imperforate Hymen — *"Have you noticed heaviness or abdominal pain every month? Have you ever had a genital exam before?"*

Androgen Insensitivity Syndrome (AIS) — *"Has anyone in your family ever mentioned concerns about your gender or development when you were born?"*

Mullerian Agenesis — *"Has a doctor ever told you that your uterus or parts of your reproductive system are underdeveloped?"*

Prolactinoma — *"Have you ever experienced any weight gain? Nipple discharge? Headaches? Vision problems?"*

Thyroid — *"Do you ever feel hot or cold when others don't? Have you ever experienced any constipation?"*

Name / Age

PC - Empathy

SOCRATES-------------------Impact

LMP

Any hx of headaches

Any visual field defects

SIGN POST DDx H A M P T P

D G P E G S

M G O S hx

P A M H U G S F O S S

|

S A D

Primary Amenorrhea (Continued)

imperforate Hymen, AIS, Mullerian Agenesis, Prolactinoma, Thyroid, Pregnancy

H A M P T P

<u>Pregnancy</u> — *"If I may ask, are you sexually active? If yes, do you think you could be pregnant? Have you checked?"*

Name / Age
PC - Empathy

SOCRATES—-------------------Impact
LMP

Any hx of headaches

Any visual field defects

DDx **H A M P T P**
D G P E G S

M G O S hx

P A M H U G S F O S S
|
S A D

Primary Amenorrhea (Continued)

Pt has never had a period

SOCRATES + **MGOS**

"Just to make sure there's nothing serious going on."

"Secondary sexual characteristics present?" If ***NO***:

Developmental Delay, Gonadal Agenesis, Pituitary Adenoma, Exercise, Genetics, Sugar

D G P E G S

DDx: *"I'd like to ask you a few questions to rule out other causes."*

Developmental Delay — *"Do you know when your mom had her period? Do you have sisters? How about their age of menarche?"*

Gonadal Agenesis — *"Do you have any f/hx of reproductive diseases or endocrine disorders?"*

Pituitary Adenoma — *"Have you noticed any changes in your vision? Any blurriness? Difficulty in your visual field? Have you experienced any headaches? Any weight gain?"*

Exercise (Functional Hypothalamic Amenorrhea) — *"How often do you engage in physical activity? Have you noticed any change in appetite? in weight?"*

Name / Age

PC - Empathy

SOCRATES-------------------Impact

LMP

Any hx of headaches

Any visual field defects

DDx **H A M P T P**

D G P E G S

M G O S hx

P A M H U G S F O S S

|

S A D

Primary Amenorrhea (Continued)

"Secondary sexual characteristics present?" If ***NO*****:**

Developmental Delay, Gonadal Agenesis, Pituitary Adenoma, Exercise, Genetics, Sugar

D G P E G S

<u>Genetics</u> – (Eg. Turner syn) — *"Any f/hx of genetic disorders? Do you have certain features like short stature, webbed neck, leg swelling, or wide-spaced nipples?"*

<u>Sugar</u> (Diabetic Mellitus) — *"Have you noticed that you have been peeing a lot? Have you been thirsty a lot? Have you been diagnosed with diabetes? Any f/hx of diabetes?"*

Name / Age

PC - Empathy

SOCRATES—-------------------Impact

LMP

Any hx of headaches

Any visual field defects

SIGN POST DDx H A M P T P

D G P E G S

M G O S hx

P A M H U G S F O S S

S A D

Secondary Amenorrhea

SOCRATES + *"LMP? Any chance that you may be pregnant? Have you checked?* + **MGOS** hx.

"Just to make sure there's nothing serious going on."

Pit A/Prolactinoma
Exercise/Endocrine
Gonads Related
Sheehan's Syndrome
Cushing's Syndrome
Asherman's Syndrome
Anorexia Nervosa
Medications

P E G S C A A M

DDx: *"I'd like to ask you a few questions to rule out other causes."*

Pituitary Adenoma/Prolactinoma — *"Have you noticed any changes in your vision? Any blurriness? Any difficulty seeing objects in your periphery? Have you experienced any headaches? Any weight gain? Any nipple discharge?"*

Exercise/Endocrine — *"How often do you engage in physical activity? Have you noticed any change in appetite? in weight?"*

Gonads Related – (PCOs/POI) Ask '**OHIA**' for PCOs (Obesity, hirsutism, infertility, acne/amenorrhea) for POI — *"Have you ever experienced hot flashes/night sweats? Do you have a family hx of early menopause?"*

Name / Age

PC - Empathy

SOCRATES---------------------**Impact**

LMP

Headaches

Visual Field Defects

Virilization (Have you noticed male pattern hair growth or deepening of voice

DDx **P E G S C A A M**

M G O S hx

P A M H U G S F O S S

|

S A D

Secondary Amenorrhea (Continued)

Pit A/Prolactinoma
Exercise/Endocrine
Gonads Related
Sheehan's Syndrome
Cushing's Syndrome
Asherman's Syndrome
Anorexia Nervosa
Medications

P E G S C A A M

Sheehan's Syndrome — *"Have you ever had any major surgery? Any hx of decreased blood supply to the brain?"*

Cushing's Syndrome — *"Have you noticed any weight gain, particularly on your tummy, back of neck, and face?"*

Asherman's Syndrome — *"Any hx of gynecological procedures? Ever had a D&C?"*

Anorexia Nervosa — *"Have you been restricting your food intake? Do you have a fear of gaining weight?"*

Medication — *"Are you on any medications?"*

Name / Age

PC - Empathy

SOCRATES———————————**Impact**

LMP

Headaches

Visual Field Defects

Virilization (Have you noticed male pattern hair growth or deepening of voice

SIGN POST DDx **P E G S C A A M**

M G O S hx

P A M H U G S F O S S

|

S A D

Vaginal Bleeding

SOCRATES → Ask **BBL**

"Just to make sure there's nothing serious going on."

Fibroid Polyps / Endometriosis/Ad / EP / Trauma/IUD/FB / Cushing's Syn / CAH / HypoT/ HyperP / Bleeding ds / Malignancy / Medications / Infection

F E E T Endo B M M I

DDx: *"I'd like to ask you a few questions to rule out other causes."*

<u>Fibroid Polyps/ Endometriosis/Adenomyosis</u> — *"Any abdominal pain?"* Ask about sexual hx *"Any painful intercourse? Do you experience heaviness/pressure or mass on your abdomen? Do you experience painful defecation?"*

<u>Ectopic Pregnancy</u> — *"When was your last menstrual period? Do you think you could be pregnant? Have you checked?"*

<u>Trauma/IUD/FB</u> — *"Did you hurt yourself? Any chance there was a foreign body placed near or around your private parts? Do you have an IUD inserted?"*

<u>Cushing's Syndrome</u> — *"Have you noticed any weight gain, particularly on your tummy, back of neck, and face?"*

Name / Age

PC - Empathy

SOCRATES—-------------------**Impact**

LMP

Is she stable?

Dizzy/Faint

Is she pregnant? (ask LMP)

Ass. pain-EP

Post-coital bleeding?

DDx **Feet Endo BMMI**

Bleeding ds - **BBL**

Infection - Cervicitis/Vaginitis/PID

M G O S hx

P A M H U G S F O S S

|

S A D

Vaginal Bleeding (Continued)

Fibroid Polyps, Endometriosis/Ad, EP, Trauma/IUD/FB, Cushing's Syn, CAH, HypoT/ HyperP, Bleeding ds, Malignancy, Medications, Infection

F E E T Endo B M M I

Congenital Adrenal Hyperplasia — *"Have you ever noticed any deepening of voice? Unusual body hair growth? Acne? Early puberty?"*

Hypothyroidism — *"Do they feel cold when others don't?"*

HyperProlactin – (Prolactinoma) — *"Have you ever experienced any weight gain? Nipple discharge? Headaches? Vision problems?"*

Bleeding Issues - ask **BBL**

Malignancy — *"Have you noticed any weight loss? Any night sweats? Any f/hx of cancer?"*

Medications — *"Are you on any medications?"*

Infections — *"Any hx of fever? Any vaginal irritation? Any d/c? (*If yes, ask **COCA-b**) *Any hx of UTIs?"*

Name / Age

PC - Empathy

SOCRATES—-------------------**Impact**

LMP

Is she stable?

Dizzy/Faint

Is she pregnant? (ask LMP)

Ass. pain-EP

Post-coital bleeding?

SIGN POST DDx **Feet Endo BMMI**

Bleeding ds - **BBL**

Infection - Cervicitis/Vaginitis/PID

M G O S hx

P A M H U G S F O S S

S A D

Vaginal Bleeding in First Trimester (T1-T2)

SOCRATES + LMP

"Just to make sure there's nothing serious going on."

Bleeding ds, EP, Abortion, Rh factor, Molar preg, Trauma

B E A R M T

DDx: *"I'd like to ask you a few questions to rule out other causes."*

Bleeding ds — Ask **BBL**

Ectopic Pregnancy — *"Did you ever get your U/S done? Is there associated abdominal pain?"*

Abortion — *"Has the bleeding been heavy or accompanied by clots? Have you ever had an abortion before?"*

Rh Factor — *"Do you know what your blood type is? Have you received Rh immunoglobulin (RhoGAM) in any previous pregnancies or after any miscarriages?"*

Molar Preg — *"Have you experienced excessive nausea or vomiting? Did you notice a rapid abdominal growth? Did your U/S after pregnancy show any abnormalities? Did your healthcare provider mention that you have unusually high BhCG levels in your blood?"*

Trauma — *"Any chance that you hurt yourself or had any trauma?"*

Name / Age

PC - Empathy

SOCRATES-------------------**Impact**

LMP

Is she stable?

Dizzy/faint

Any associated pain?

(signs of EP/ Trauma)

DDx **B E A R M T**

Bleeding ds - **BBL**

Recurrent losses? → DDX **A C U E**

M G O S hx

P A M H U G S F O S S

|

S A D

Vaginal Bleeding in First Trimester (T1-T2) (Continued)

Bleeding ds, EP, Abortion, Rh factor, Molar preg, Trauma

B E A R M T

Recurrent losses? If yes →

APAS, Chromosomal Abnormality, Uterine Structural Abnormality, Endocrine

A C U E

Antiphospholipid Antibody Syndrome (APAS) — *"Have you had any previous miscarriages or pregnancy issues? Do you have a previous or f/hx of blood clotting disorder? Any hx of severe leg pain/ swelling?"*

Chromosomal abnormalities — *"Any hx of genetic or chromosomal abnormalities in your family?"*

Uterine Structural Abnormality — *"Have you ever been diagnosed with uterine fibroids? Any structural issues with your uterus? Have you had any surgeries such as D&C or a myomectomy?"*

Endocrine — *"Any hx of hormonal issues in the past? Have you been diagnosed with DM? Do you ever feel cold when others don't?"*

Name / Age

PC - Empathy

SOCRATES—------------------**Impact**

LMP

Is she stable?

Dizzy/faint

Any associated pain?

(signs of EP/ Trauma)

DDx **B E A R M T**

Bleeding ds - **BBL**

Recurrent losses? → DDX **A C U E**

M G O S hx

P A M H U G S F O S S

|

S A D

Vaginal Bleeding in Third Trimester (T3)

SOCRATES + LMP

"Just to make sure there's nothing serious going on."

Placenta Previa, Abruptio Placenta, Trauma, Infection, Bleeding ds, Uterine Rupture, Tumor

P A T in B U T

DDx: *"I'd like to ask you a few questions to rule out other causes."*

Placenta Previa (PP) — Pt will indicate **painless** vaginal bleeding. *"Have you had any U/S done during pregnancy that has indicated the position of the placenta?"*

Abruptio Placenta (AP) — Pt will indicate **painful** vaginal bleeding. *"Have you noticed any changes to the baby's movts? Do you feel it kicking?"*

Trauma — *"Any chance that you hurt yourself or had any trauma?"*

Infection — *"Any hx of fever? Any vaginal irritation? Any d/c? (*If yes, ask **COCA-b**) *Any hx of UTIs?"*

Uterine Rupture — *"Did you ever have a cesarean section before? Was it a classic incision? Any hx of surgeries on your uterus?"*

Tumor — *"Any hx of cancer? Any weight loss? Any lumps or bumps on their body?"*

Name / Age

PC - Empathy

SOCRATES--------------------**Impact**

LMP

Is she stable?

Dizzy/faint

Hx of trauma

Pain

DDx **P A T in B U T**

Bleeding ds - **BBL**

M G O S hx

P A M H U G S F O S S

S A D

Vaginal Bleeding - Elderly

SOCRATES + LMP + **BBL**

"Just to make sure there's nothing serious going on."

Bleeding issues, Endometrial CA, Atrophic Vaginitis, Trauma, Sexual Abuse, Cervix Carcinoma

B E A T S - cervix

DDx: *"I'd like to ask you a few questions to rule out other causes."*

Bleeding Issues — Ask **BBL**

Endometrial Carcinoma — Ask about constitutional s/s and **COLD NUT**

Atrophic Vaginitis — *"Have you noticed any itching or burning in your vaginal area? Do you experience any discomfort during intercourse?"*

Trauma/Sexual Abuse — *"Any chance that you hurt yourself or had any trauma? Are you in a relationship? Do you feel safe in your relationship? Did you ever have sexual intercourse where you felt uncomfortable?"*

Cervix Carcinoma — *"Have you noticed any weight loss/ night sweats/ fever? Any hx of cancer? Any family hx of cancer?"*

Ask sexual hx.

Name / Age

PC - Empathy

SOCRATES——------------------**Impact**

LMP

Constitutional s/s

- Weight loss
- Fever
- Night sweats
- Hx and f/hx of cancer

DDx B E A T S - cervix

Bleeding ds - **BBL**

Endometrial Carcinoma - constitutional s/s + **COLD NUT**

Menopause hx - VU FIDL B B

M G O S hx

P A M H U G S F O S S

|

S A D

Polycystic Ovarian Syndrome (POS)

Pt may come with complaints of menstrual irregularity or hirsutism/ acne.

Obesity, Hirsutism, Infertility, Acne, DM, Acanthosis Nigricans

SOCRATES + O H I A D A

Remember Rotterdam Criteria –

- Irregular menstruation > 6 months
- Increased testosterone (s/s of acne and hirsutism)
- u/s ovary → PCO

SIGN POST *"Just to make sure there's nothing serious going on."*

CAH, Cushing's Syn, Hyperprolactinemia, Hypothyroidism

C C H H

SIGN POST DDx: *"I'd like to ask you a few questions to rule out other causes."*

<u>Congenital Adrenal Hyperplasia</u> — *"Have you ever noticed any deepening of voice? Unusual body hair growth? Acne? Early puberty?"*

<u>Cushing's Syndrome</u> — *"Have you noticed any weight gain, particularly on your tummy, back of neck, and face?"*

<u>Hyperprolactinemia</u> — *"Have you ever experienced any weight gain? Nipple d/c? Headaches? Vision problems?"*

<u>Hypothyroidism</u> — *"Do they feel cold when others don't?"*

Name / Age

PC - Empathy

SOCRATES—-------------------**Impact**

Associated s/s- **OHIA DA**

LMP

Any hx of headaches

Any visual field defects

SIGN POST DDx C C H H

M G O S hx

P A M H U G S F O S S

S A D

Pelvic Pain

"Just to make sure there's nothing serious going on."

ovarian Torsion
rupture of Ovarian Cyst
Ectopic Pregnancy
PID
Abuse/Trauma

T O E P A

DDx: *"I'd like to ask you a few questions to rule out other causes."*

<u>Ovarian Torsion/Rupture of Ovarian Cyst</u>
Sudden onset, one-sided severe pain.

<u>Ectopic Pregnancy</u> — Ask about LMP.
"Did you ever get your U/S done? Is there associated vaginal bleeding / or abdominal pain?"

<u>PID</u> — Ask sexual hx - number of partners/ smoking hx/ hx of STIs/ practicing safe sex/ IUDs/ fever/ vaginal d/c.

Name / Age
PC - Empathy

SOCRATES—-------------------**Impact**

LMP

Rule out Ectopic Pregnancy

Trauma/Bleeding
Is Pt stable?
Dizzy/Faint?
Abuse/Trauma

DDx T O E P A

(Also, check DDx for abdominal pain in GIT - **AIRPAD)**

M G O S hx

P A M H U G S F O S S
|
S A D

Infertility

SOCRATES + Infertility hx

- ↓35 yrs → 12 months duration
- 35 yrs - 40 yrs → 6 months duration
- ↑40 yrs → right away

SIGN POST *"Just to make sure there's nothing serious going on."*

Endocrine Pituitary Ovarian Uterine

E P O U + genetics

SIGN POST DDx: *"I'd like to ask you a few questions to rule out other causes."*

Endocrine — Ask about thyroid, DM, and adrenals.

Pituitary — Ask about pituitary adenomas/ prolactinomas/ Sheehan's syndrome. *"Do you get any headaches? Have you noticed any visual disturbances? Any nipple d/c? Have you ever had any complications in your previous delivery or surgery?"*

Ovarian — Ask **OHIA** for PCOs, for POI. *"Have you ever experienced hot flashes/night sweats? Do you have a family hx of early menopause?"*

Uterine — Ask about Endometriosis fibroids, Asherman's syndrome, PID, Adenomyosis, IUDs, and Structural abnormality.

Name / Age

PC - Empathy

SOCRATES——-----------------Impact

LMP

Headaches

Visual field defects

Ask for detailed hx of **MGOS**

Ask about DM/ Prolactin/Thyroid

SIGN POST causes E P O U + genetics

M G O S hx

P A M H U G S F O S S

S A D

Infertility (Continued)

Endocrine Pituitary Ovarian Uterine

E P O U + genetics

Genetics — (E.g. Kartagener's, Kallman's, Turner) *"Any hx of genetic chromosomal abnormalities in your family?"*

Name / Age
PC - Empathy

SOCRATES—-------------------Impact

LMP

Headaches

Visual field defects

Ask for detailed hx of **MGOS**

Ask about DM/ Prolactin/Thyroid

SIGN POST causes E P O U + genetics

M G O S hx

P A M   H U G S   F O S S

S A D

Hirsutism

"Just to make sure there's nothing serious going on."

hypoThyroid, Adrenal Adenoma, PRL, PCOs, Ovarian Adenoma, Steroids, Cushing's Syn, CAH

T A P P O S C C

DDx: *"I'd like to ask you a few questions to rule out other causes."*

Hypothyroid — *"Do you feel cold when others don't?"*

s/s of ↑ androgens – ↑Muscle bulk, male pattern balding, deepened voice, clitoromegaly.

(PRL) Prolactinoma — *"Any hx of weight gain? Any nipple d/c? Headache? Visual field defects?"*

PCOs — Ask questions about **OHIA DA**.

Steroids — *"Are you taking any steroids lately?"*

Cushing's Syndrome — *"Have you noticed any weight gain, particularly on your tummy, back of neck, and face?"*

Congenital Adrenal Hyperplasia — *"Have you ever noticed any deepening of voice? Unusual body hair growth? Acne? Early puberty?"*

Name / Age

PC - Empathy

SOCRATES--------------------Impact

LMP

Sudden onset

Deepened voice/ male pattern balding.

DDx T A P P O S C C

M G O S hx

P A M H U G S F O S S

S A D

Vaginal Discharge

SOCRATES + **COCA-b +**
"Is it associated with: itching, fever, lesions on genitalia, ulcers on genitalia or mouth, rash, abdominal pain, or hx of UTIs?"

"I flura u"

MGOS
↳ Ask about Risky Behavior:

MSM
Age of Intercourse
multiple Sexual partners
unprotected Sex
Hx of STIs
IUD

M A S S Hx I

Remember →May need to <u>Report</u>
→Treat sexual partners
→Admit if PID

Name / Age

PC - Empathy

SOCRATES—-------------------Impact

Associated s/s - **I Flura U**

COCA-B + LMP

CONFIDENTIALITY

M G O S hx

+ Risky Behaviour - **"MASSHi"**

If adolescents, ask **HEADSS**

P A M H U G S F O S S

|

S A D

Preeclampsia

Information at the station will indicate that the pt is pregnant with high blood pressure, and protein in urine. If it comes with urine analysis: *"I have your results and would like to discuss them with you. I'd like to ask you a few questions first since it's the first time we are meeting."*

"Just to make sure there's nothing serious going on."

Chest Pain
Headaches
Urinary Changes
Drooping of Face - in BE FAST
HELLP syndrome

C H U D + hellp

BE FAST stands for Balance, Eyesight changes, Facial Drooping, Arm weakness, Speech/Swallowing difficulty, Time to call 911 *"Did you notice any issues with balance/or with your eyes? (*Blurring of vision) *Any dropping of face, weakness of arm/leg, difficulty swallowing or speaking?*" (If all positive go to ER → Alert stroke code)

HELLP Syndrome — *"Do you notice any bruises on your body? Any yellow discoloration on your skin? Any dark urine? Pale stools?"*

Preeclampsia RF → *"First time pregnant? First baby with this partner? Previous hx of HTN/ DM/ Stillbirth?"*

Name / Age

PC - Empathy

SOCRATES——-------------------Impact

LMP

Ask C H U D + help

Preeclampsia RF

Pregnancy Hx - **PPF Chun VBL**

+ **ABCDE**

M G O S hx

P A M H U G S F O S S

S A D

Abortion

Possible counselling station - Pt may request an abortion / or the station can also present as breaking bad news.

Confidentiality

Pregnancy questions - **PPF Chun VBL**

- Ask about mood
- Ask about family support

Rule out contradictions for abortion -

- Ectopic Pregnancy
- Adrenal Failure
- Ambivalence

Name / Age

PC - Empathy

SOCRATES—-------------------Impact

LMP

🚩 *Is she stable?*

Dizzy/faint

Any associated pain?

(signs of EP/ Trauma)

Pregnancy Hx - **PPF Chun VBL**

\+ 🚩 **ABCDE**

M G O S hx

P A M H U G S F O S S

|

S A D

Menopause

Possible counselling station.

SOCRATES

+ Vu Fidl BB

- Osteoporosis - Check RF (details on next page) **FELS R MAD**
- Can also ask RF for endometrial carcinoma - **COLDNUT**

Name / Age

PC - Empathy

SOCRATES—-------------------Impact

Menopause hx **Vu FidL BB**

RF: **FELS R MAD**

Can also ask **COLD NUT**

M G O S hx

P A M H U G S F O S S

|

S A D

Osteoporosis

Pt can present with f# / fall / decrease height / BMD results.

"Just to make sure there's nothing serious going on."

f/hx of f# | Endocrine | LBW | Smoking | RA | Malabsorption | Alcohol | Drugs

F E L S R M A D

RF: *"I'd like to ask you a few questions to rule out any risk factors."*

Family hx of f# — *"Any family hx of f#?"*

Endocrine (DM, T, PTH) — *"Do you have any medical conditions like DM? Do you feel like you need to pee a lot? Or drink a lot? Have you ever felt cold or hot when others don't? Any hx of kidney stones? Constipation?"*

LBW *(Low body weight)* — *"Do you feel like your body weight is ideal?"*

Smoking — *"Do you smoke? Since when have you been smoking? How many cigarettes per day?"*

Rheumatoid Arthritis — *"Any past medical hx of any autoimmune conditions? Do you have any joint pain? Any nodules on your fingers? Any deformities of your hands?"*

Malabsorption — Ask about celiac disease, hx of gastrectomy or intestinal resection, and IBD.

Alcohol — *"Do you drink alcohol? How often? How many glasses a day?"*

Name / Age

PC - Empathy

SOCRATES—-------------------Impact

Pain/ swelling/ fever/ warmth

(signs of septic arthritis)

RF **F E L S R M A D**

F R A X - assess risk

MGOS hx + Menopause hx

P A M H U G S F O S S

S A D

Osteoporosis (Continued)

f/hx of f# · Endocrine · LBW · Smoking · RA · Malabsorption · Alcohol · Drugs

F E L S R M A D

Drugs — *"Are you on any medications?"* Drugs causing osteoporosis include steroids, androgen deprivation therapy, anti-estrogens, chemotherapy, and heparin.

Name / Age

PC - Empathy

SOCRATES———————————Impact

Pain/ swelling/ fever/ warmth

(signs of septic arthritis)

SIGN POST

RF **F E L S R M A D**

F R A X - assess risk

MGOS hx + Menopause hx

P A M H U G S F O S S

|

S A D

Cardiovascular/ Respiratory System

How to organise yourself before entering the station + KEY **40**

Chest Pain. **44**

Chest Pain - Myocardial Infarction **46**

Chest Pain - Aortic Dissection **47**

Chest Pain - Pericarditis **48**

Chest Pain - GERD **49**

Chest Pain - Aortic Stenosis. **50**

Chest Pain - Pulmonary Embolism **52**

Chest Pain - Pneumothorax **53**

Heart Racing **55**

Atrial Fibrillation (AF). **57**

Hypertension **59**

Syncope **61**

Congestive Heart Failure (CHF) **63**

Deep Vein Thrombosis (DVT) **64**

Peripheral Artery Disease (PAD) **66**

Cough **68**

Hemoptysis **69**

Asthma **71**

COPD **73**

How to organise yourself before entering the station

Before entering the station, you will have under two minutes to read the prompt and jot down notes in your booklet.

These notes should focus on key information you'll need to remember while taking the history from the standardized participant (SP). The SP is an actor trained to portray a specific medical condition or scenario. Their purpose is to interact with you and allow the physician examiner (PE) to observe and assess your performance.

The booklet provided is rectangular, about half the size of an A4 sheet. It contains blank sheets for your notes, as well as candidate code stickers, which you'll need to hand over to the examiner before starting each station.

Given the time constraints and anxiety during the station, these notes can serve as a valuable guide to help you complete a thorough history.

Therefore, it is essential to practice responding to prompts and mastering the '2-minute drill' regularly to achieve your best results.

HOW TO PRACTICE :

For practice purposes, folding an A4 sheet in half works well to simulate the booklet.

Hence this book is divided into two columns:

Left column	**Right column**
Contains a breakdown of the mnemonics and the questions you may need to ask.	Notes to write in your booklet as part of your 2-minute drill, often including mnemonics that make the best use of your time and help you recall essential steps efficiently!

These structured notes will provide a clear and concise roadmap to ensure you stay focused and efficient during the station.

The KEY

Knock on the door, Walk in, Wear a smile, Greet the examiner, and hand the candidate code, *"Hi, here's my candidate code."*
Sanitize your hands and simultaneously:

Introduce yourself to the standardized participant (SP):
"Hello, I am Dr___ and I will be your physician today. May I know your name and age, please? How would you like to be addressed? That's great!

"Is it okay if I sit down and take a few notes?"

PC: Presenting Complaints
"What brings you in here today?"
Listen to the patient. It is important to express **Empathy.**
"I am sorry to hear that. That must be quite distressing."

"Okay, so I would like to ask you a few questions and do a physical exam after and we will figure out a treatment plan for you today!"

SOCRATES-B: For conditions with other symptoms SOCRATES-B can still be used.

- site: *"Where is the pain? Can you point at it?"*
- onset: *"Was it gradual or sudden in onset?"*
- character: *"What kind of pain is it? Is it a dull pain or a sharp pain?"*
- radiate: *"Does the pain radiate anywhere?"*
- associated symptoms: *"Any associated symptoms?"*
- time: *"Is the pain constant or intermittent?"*
- exacerbating factor: *"Does anything relieve the pain or make it worse?"*
- severity: *"On a scale from 1-10, how would you rate the pain? 10 being the worst."*
- before: *"Have you had this before?"*

Not every P/C involves pain. Some complaints may just require 'o-ate' onset associated s/s, time, and exacerbating/ relieving factors.

COCA-b: For any vomiting/discharge/sputum/stool/urine.
Colour, **O**dor, **C**onsistency, **A**mount, **B**lood (If yes for blood, ask **BBL**)

BBL — (if pt complains of bleeding), stands for :

- Blood thinners – *"Are you on blood thinners?"*
- Bloody Diarrhea – *"Do you bruise easily or bleed easily?"*
- Liver Disease — *"Any hx of liver disease?"*

Impact: *"How are you coping with this?"*

DDX: Differentials for the condition given for each condition.

SIGNPOST: This symbol means you have to signpost! A signpost is an introductory statement. This is to introduce your segment of questions so the examiner is aware of your line of questioning.

E.g.: DDx - means you have to place an introductory statement before asking for differentials: *"I am going to ask a few questions to rule out any other causes."*

Red flags: This is for conditions we need to rule out right away as they may require urgent attention.

PAM HUGS FOSS: stands for:

- Past medical hx: *"Since this is the first time we are meeting, do you have any past medical conditions that I should know about? Or that you have been treated for?"*
- Allergies: *"Do you have any allergies?"*
- Medications: *"Are you on any medications? What are the medications? Are you adherent with your medications? What is the dosage?"*
- Hospitalization/Surgery: *"Have you ever been hospitalized before? Any surgeries done before?"*
- Urinary changes: *"Have you noticed changes in your urine?"*
- GIT changes: *"Have you noticed any changes in your bowel habits?"*
- SAD- **S**moking/**A**lcohol/Recreational **D**rugs:
    - *"Do you smoke? How many cigarettes a day? For how long? Have you ever thought about quitting?"*
    - *"Do you drink alcohol? How often?"*
    - *"Have you done any recreational drugs? What have you used? How do you take it? Do you sniff or inject? Do you share needles?"*
- Family history: *"Any family history of any medical conditions?"* Specific medical conditions you are concerned about.
- Occupation: *"If I may ask, what do you do for a living?"*
- Social: *"May I know about your living conditions? Who do you live with?"*
- Support: *"Do you have any family around? Are they supportive? That's good to know."*

Mnemonics for system questions:
Cardiovascular/Respiratory:

SOB: Shortness **O**f **B**reath

- *" Do you have difficulty speaking?"*
- *"Have you ever had to go to the hospital because of it?"*
- *"Did you ever turn blue?"*
- *"How many pillows do you use?"*
- *"Do you ever wake up gasping for air?"*

St. SoHeCo AbViLoC

- Sweating – *"Did you notice any sweating?"*
- chest Tightness — *"Are you feeling any chest tightness?"*
- **SOB -** (ask the 5 questions from above)
- Heart racing — *"Do you feel your heart is beating too fast or skipping a beat? Any palpitations?"*
- Cough — *"Is it a dry cough or do you get sputum with it?* (if yes, ask **COCA b**) *"No sputum? – What kind of cough, what does it sound like? Is it a barking cough? Any chest sounds like a wheeze or a whistle?"*
- Abdominal Pain — *"Is it associated with meals?* (mesenteric angina)
- blurry Vision — *"Any blurring of vision?"*
- Loss of consciousness — *"Any loss of consciousness? Did you black out? Fall? Get hurt? Did you have anyone there with you?"*
- Calf Pain — *"Any calf swelling? Any leg pain? Any weakness? Numbness? Loss of sensation? Any pain after walking?*

St. SoHeCo AbViLoC **fetraSic DES has Brejt** (Extended version)

- Fever — *"Any fever?"*
- Travel hx — *"Any hx of travel? Or long flight?"*
- Sick contacts — *"Any sick contacts?*

- Diet — *"How's your diet? Do you eat healthy? Enjoy a lot of fast food?"*
- Exercise — *"Do you exercise? How many blocks can you walk? Previously?*
- Stress — *"Have there been any stressors in your life lately?"*

- heartburn — *"Any heartburn?"*
- acidic taste — *"Any acidic or sour taste in your mouth?"*
- swallowing — *"Do you have difficulty swallowing?/or painful swallowing?"* (Esophageal spasm/Esophagitis)

- Blisters/rash — *"Any blisters or rashes on your skin?"* (Herpes Zoster)
- runny nose — *"Any runny nose?"* (URTI)
- runny eyes — *"Any red eyes?"* (URTI)
- Jt swelling/pain — *"Any joint swelling?"* (Autoimmune /Rheumatology/ SLE)

Chest Pain

SOCRATES - **Site of pain!** *"Can you point to where the pain is?"*

SIGN POST *"Just to make sure there's nothing serious going on."*

MI AD Pericarditis GERD AS PTX PE Costochondritis CHF

m a p g a p p c

SIGN POST DDx: *"I'd like to ask you a few questions to rule out other causes."*

Myocardial Infarction (MI) — Pt complains of substernal pain, ↑ on exertion, possibly radiating to the left arm, SOB, relieved by NTG/aspirin (angina).

Aortic Dissection (AD) — Pt complains of tearing/sharp pain that radiates to the back. May have ass. dyspnea/ numbness.

Pericarditis — Pt pain decreases when leaning forward & worsens when lying down.

GERD — Pt complains of a sour taste in their mouth/ heartburn and chronic cough.

Aortic Stenosis (AS) — Pt complains of pain or SOB on exertion/palpitations/dizziness, lightheadedness or syncope/ ↓ exercise tolerance.

Pneumothorax (PTX) — Pt has hx of lung disease, trauma, or smoking. Ass. with SOB, sharp pain worse with breathing.

Name / Age

PC - Empathy

SOCRATES———————Impact

Associated trauma

Dizzy/ faint

CVS Hx - St SoheCo AbviLoC

diet/exercise/stress

SIGN POST DDx m a p g a p pc

Last meal? (In case it's an emergency)

P A M H U G S F O S S

↓ ↪Cialis/Viagra |

HTN **S A D**
DM
Cholesterol
Triggers?
Stress?

Chest Pain (Continued)

MI AD Pericarditis GERD AS PTX PE Costochondritis CHF

m a p g a p p c

Pulmonary Embolism (PE) — Pt has hx of DVT/leg pain/immobility/recent surgery/ cancer hx/ on OCPs. Ass. with **SOB**, pink frothy sputum.

Costochondritis — *"Does the pain get worse when you press on your chest around the ribs/breastbone? Does the pain get worse with breathing/coughing or twisting?"*

Exacerbation of Congestive Heart Failure (CHF) — Ass. with SOB, eye puffiness, ankle swelling, Hx of heart disease.

Name / Age
PC - Empathy

SOCRATES—-------------------Impact

Associated trauma

Dizzy/ faint

CVS Hx - St SoheCo AbviLoC

diet/exercise/stress

SIGN POST DDx m a p g a p pc

Last meal? (In case it's an emergency)

P A M H U G S F O S S

↓ ↪Cialis/Viagra |

HTN
DM
Cholesterol
Triggers?
Stress?

S A D

Chest Pain - Myocardial Infarction

SOCRATES —

- Sharp Substernal Pain *(May radiate to left arm)*
- Pain on Exertion
- Relieved by rest/NTG

MI AD Pericarditis GERD AS PTX PE Costochondritis CHF

m a p g a p p c

DDx: *"I'd like to ask you a few questions to rule out other causes."*

Myocardial Infarction (MI) — Pt complains of substernal pain, ↑ on exertion, possibly radiating to the left arm, SOB, relieved by NTG/aspirin (angina).

Mgx-
C — 12 lead ECG
C — **C**ardiac Markers
C — Urgent **C**ardiac Consult
C — Send to **C**ath lab

Morphine O2 NTG Aspirin Heparin

M O N A - H

Name / Age
PC - Empathy

SOCRATES—-------------------Impact

Associated trauma

Dizzy/ faint

CVS Hx - St SoheCo AbviLoC

diet/exercise/stress

DDx m a p g a p pc

P A M H U G S F O S S

↓ ↪Cialis/Viagra |

HTN
DM
Cholesterol
Triggers?
Stress?

S A D

Mgx - M O N A - H

Chest Pain - Aortic Dissection

SOCRATES —

- Sharp tearing pain - radiates to the back.
- Pain can be elsewhere depending on the area with compromised blood supply due to AD. May have associated dyspnea/ numbness.
- Can be associated with decreased urine output, abdominal pain or flank pain.

"Just to make sure there's nothing serious going on."

MI AD Pericarditis GERD AS PTX PE Costochondritis CHF

m a p g a p p c

DDx: *"I'd like to ask you a few questions to rule out other causes."*

RF *"I'd like to ask you a few questions to rule out any risk factors."*

"Any hx of hypertension? Any family hx of connective tissue disorder? Do you have long arms and long fingers as compared to others? Any heart conditions or congenital heart diseases? Any vascular diseases? Any hx of trauma?"

Name / Age

PC - Empathy

SOCRATES——-------------------Impact

Associated trauma

Dizzy/ faint

CVS Hx - St SoheCo AbviLoC

diet/exercise/stress

DDx m a p g a p p c

Marfan's Syn Ehler Danlos Syn Syphilis Trauma Takayasu's Arteritis

RF: HTN M E ♥ S T T

Heart
-CoArctation of Aorta
-Bicuspid valves

P A M H U G S F O S S

↓ ↪Cialis/Viagra |

HTN
DM
Cholesterol
Triggers?
Stress?

S A D

Last meal?

Chest Pain - Pericarditis

SOCRATES —

- Sharp pain, worse on lying down.
- Pain gets better with leaning forward.
- Associated with SOB, fatigue, and palpitations.

SIGN POST *"Just to make sure there's nothing serious going on."*

MI AD Pericarditis GERD AS PTX PE Costochondritis CHF

m a p g a p p c

SIGN POST DDx: *"I'd like to ask you a few questions to rule out other causes."*

Prior Viral Infection Previous MI hypoThyroidism Hydralazine Autoimmune

V mi t h a

Previous Viral Infection — *"Any hx of fever/flu-like symptoms?"*

Previous Myocardial infarction — *"Any hx of heart disease? MI? Post - CABG?"*

Hypothyroidism — *"Do you feel cold when others don't? Did you notice any unintentional weight gain? Do you have a hx of constipation?"*

Autoimmune — *"Any past medical hx of autoimmune conditions?"*

Name / Age

PC - Empathy

SOCRATES--------------------Impact

Associated trauma

Dizzy/ faint

CVS Hx - St SoheCo AbviLoC

diet/exercise/stress

SIGN POST DDx m a p g a p pc

(Can address possible causes)-

V m i t h a

P A M H U G S F O S S

|

S A D

Chest Pain - GERD

SOCRATES —

- Chest pain at night, worse on lying down.
- Chest pain after meals
- Hx of heartburn/sour taste in mouth/chronic cough.

"Just to make sure there's nothing serious going on."

Weight Loss, Bleeding, persistent Vomiting, difficulty Swallowing, F/hx of Cancer

W B V S F

Angina, PUD, Gastritis, Achalasia, Malignancy, Esophagitis

DDx AP GAME

DDx: *"I'd like to ask you a few questions to rule out other causes."*

Angina — *"Any hx heart disease? Is there pain on exertion? relieved by rest?"*

Peptic Ulcer disease (PUD) — *"Is the pain associated with eating? Does it occur on an empty stomach? Do you take any anti-inflammatory medications? Have you noticed any black tarry stools?"*

Gastritis — *"Do experience nausea, vomiting? Do you drink alcohol?"*

Name / Age

PC - Empathy

SOCRATES—-------------------Impact

W B V S F

CVS Hx - St SoheCo AbviLoC

diet/exercise/stress

DDx AP GAME

RF D G S H O P

P A M H U G S F O S S

↓

Stress?

S A D

Chest Pain - GERD (Continued)

Angina PUD Gastritis Achalasia Malignancy Esophagitis

DDx A P G A M E

Achalasia — *"Is the pain intermittent? Any difficulty swallowing?"*

Malignant — *"Any weight loss/ night sweats/ fever? Any hx of cancer or f/hx of cancer?"*

Esophagitis — *"Do you experience pain while swallowing? fever? DM? Are you on immunosuppressants?"*

Diet Gastric stasis Smoking Hernia (Hiatal) Obesity Pregnancy

RF: D G S H O P

SIGN POST RF *"I'd like to ask you a few questions to rule out any risk factors."*

RF: Do you take large meals? Late-night meals? Do you drink a lot of alcohol?/ or coffee? Do you smoke? How often? Any hx of hernia? Do you find that your weight is ideal? Could you be pregnant by any chance?"

Name / Age

PC - Empathy

SOCRATES———————Impact

W B V S F

CVS Hx - St SoheCo AbviLoC

diet/exercise/stress

SIGN POST DDx A P G A M E

RF D G S H O P

P A M H U G S F O S S

↓ (P A M): Stress?

| (H U G S): **S A D**

Chest Pain - Aortic Stenosis

Pt complains of pain on exertion/SOB on exertion/syncope.

SOCRATES
+ **SOB**? — (if yes) *"Do you have difficulty speaking? Ever had to go to the hospital because of it? Did you ever turn blue? How many pillows do you use? Do you ever wake up gasping for air?"*

SIGN POST *"Just to make sure there's nothing serious going on."*

MI AD Pericarditis GERD AS PTX PE Costochondritis CHF
m a p g a p p c

SIGN POST DDx: *"I'd like to ask you a few questions to rule out other causes."* *(Refer to Chest Pain)*

Name / Age
PC - Empathy

SOCRATES——-------------------Impact

Associated trauma

Dizzy/ faint

CVS Hx - St SoheCo AbviLoC

diet/exercise/stress

SIGN POST DDx m a p g a p p c

P A M H U G S F O S S

↓ ↪Cialis/Viagra |

S A D

HTN
DM
Cholesterol
Triggers?
Stress?

Chest Pain - Pulmonary Embolism

Pt may have hx of DVT/ leg pain/ immobility/ recent surgery/ cancer hx or/ on OCPs.

SOCRATES —

- Pain worse with breathing (pleuritic pain)
- *"Have you noticed any pink frothy sputum?"*
- **SOB?**— If yes – *"Do you have difficulty speaking? Ever had to go to the hospital because of it? Did you ever turn blue? How many pillows do you use? Do you ever wake up gasping for air?"*

SIGN POST *"Just to make sure there's nothing serious going on."*

\+ Can ask about (Well's criteria):

Edema
Alternate Δ less likely
rule out Trauma
Cancer
Hemoptysis
Immobilization
Prev hx of DVT
Surgery done within Past 4 weeks

EAT CHIPS

"Any calf swelling or leg pain? Any numbness or weakness/tingling? Any hx of long travel or flight? Any hx of cancer? Any hx of trauma? Have you experienced bloody sputum or pink frothy sputum while coughing? Have you had a recent hx of surgery or immobilization? Any previous hx of leg pain?"

Name / Age

PC - Empathy

SOCRATES---------------------Impact

Associated trauma

Dizzy/ faint

Can ask abt: EAT CHIPS

CVS Hx - St SoheCo AbviLoC

diet/exercise/stress

SIGN POST DDx map gap pc

P A M H U G S F O S S

|

S A D

Chest Pain - Pulmonary Embolism (Continued)

MI AD Pericarditis GERD AS PTX PE Costochondritis CHF

m a p g a p p c

DDx: *"I'd like to ask you a few questions to rule out other causes."*

(Refer to Chest Pain)

Name / Age

PC - Empathy

SOCRATES—------------------Impact

Associated trauma

Dizzy/ faint

Can ask abt: **E A T C H I P S**

CVS Hx - St SoheCo AbviLoC

diet/exercise/stress

DDx **m a p g a p pc**

P A M H U G S F O S S

|

S A D

Chest Pain - Pneumothorax

Pt may have a hx of lung disease, trauma, or smoking.

SOCRATES –

- Pain worse with breathing (Sharp pleuritic pain)
- Ask **SOB** + hx of trauma, smoking, and lung disease (Asthma/COPD)

"Just to make sure there's nothing serious going on."

MI AD Pericarditis GERD AS PTX PE Costochondritis CHF

m a p g a p p c

DDx: *"I'd like to ask you a few questions to rule out other causes."*

(Refer to Chest Pain)

Name / Age

PC - Empathy

SOCRATES——————-Impact

Associated trauma

Dizzy/ faint

CVS Hx - St SoheCo AbviLoC

diet/exercise/stress

DDx m a p g a p pc

P A M H U G S F O S S

|

S A D

Heart Racing

SOCRATES + CVS Hx

SIGN POST "*Just to make sure there's nothing serious going on.*"

hyperThyroidism, Arrhythmias/AS/Alcohol, Pregnancy, Panic Attack, Pheochromocytoma, Infection, Dehydration, Caffeine, Cocaine

T A P P P i D C

SIGN POST DDx: "*I'd like to ask you a few questions to rule out other causes.*"

Hyperthyroidism — "*Do you feel hot or sweaty when others don't? Have you noticed recent weight loss despite having a good appetite?*"

Arrhythmia/ Aortic Stenosis/ Alcohol (Holiday Heart) — "*Any hx of chest pain? SOB on exertion? Any hx of lightheadedness or fainting? Did you notice a decrease in exercise tolerance? Did you drink more alcohol than usual lately?*"

Pregnancy — "*When was your last menstrual period? Any chance you might be pregnant?*"

Name / Age

PC - Empathy

SOCRATES—-------------------Impact

Chest pain

Dizzy/ Faint

CVS Hx - St SoheCo AbviLoC

diet/exercise/stress

SIGN POST DDx T A P P P i D C

P A M H U G S F O S S

|

S A D

Heart Racing (Continued)

hyperThyroidism / Arrhythmias/AS/Alcohol / Pregnancy / Panic Attack / Pheochromocytoma / Infection / Dehydration / Caffeine / Cocaine

T A P P P i D C

Panic Attack — *"Are you the kind of person who is anxious a lot? Have you ever had a panic attack? Do you have symptoms of nausea, trembling, chills, choking, sweating, feeling like you might be dying or feeling out of control?"*

Pheochromocytoma — *"Any hx of pulsating headaches? Any perspiration associated with the heart racing?"*

Infection — *"Have you noticed any fever? Any red eyes?/ runny nose?/ear d/c?/ sore throat?/ cough?/ diarrhea?/ burning micturition?/neck stiffness?/ joint pain or hx of travel? Have you had any sick contacts?"*

Dehydration — *"Have you had enough fluid intake lately? Have you noticed dry lips? Sunken eyes?"*

Caffeine/Cocaine — *"Have you been drinking a lot of tea or coffee lately? How many cups? Have you ever tried any recreational drugs? Have you ever tried cocaine?"*

Name / Age

PC - Empathy

SOCRATES——------------------Impact

Chest pain

Dizzy/ Faint

CVS Hx - St SoheCo AbviLoC

diet/exercise/stress

SIGN POST DDx T A P P P i D C

P A M H U G S F O S S

|

S A D

Atrial Fibrillation (AF)

Pt may present with palpitations/ dizziness/ lightheadedness or **SOB**.

- If Palpitations → ask TAPPPID C
- If **SOB** →Ask the 5 questions.
- If dizziness/lightheadedness → *Clarify* if the room is spinning (vertigo) or lightheadedness/ fainting (syncope/cardiac).

SIGN POST *"Just to make sure there's nothing serious going on."*

New onset atrial fibrillation due to:

Pulmonary Embolism
Infection
Respiratory ds
Atrial Enlargement/Valvular ds
Thyroid
Ethanol
Sleep Apnea/
Sepsis

P I R A T E S

SIGN POST DDx: *"I'd like to ask you a few questions to rule out other causes."*

<u>Pulmonary Embolism</u> — *"**SOB?** Have you noticed any pink frothy sputum?"*

<u>Infection</u> — *"Have you noticed any fever? Any red eyes?/ runny nose?/ear d/c?/ sore throat?/ cough?/ diarrhea?/ burning micturition?/neck stiffness?/ joint pain or hx of travel? Have you had any sick contacts?"*

<u>Respiratory disease</u> — *"Have you had any respiratory diseases?"*

Name / Age

PC - Empathy

SOCRATES——------------------Impact

Chest pain

CVS Hx - St SoheCo AbviLoC

diet/exercise/stress

SIGN POST DDx **P I R A T E S**

P A M H U G S F O S S

|

S A D

Atrial Fibrillation (AF) (Continued)

Pulmonary Embolism
Infection
Respiratory ds
Atrial Enlargement/Valvular ds
Thyroid
Ethanol
Sleep Apnea/
Sepsis

P I R A T E S

Atrial Enlargement/Valvular ds — *"Any hx of heart disease? Valvular disease?"*

Thyroid — *"Do you feel hot or sweaty when others don't? Have you noticed recent weight loss despite having a good appetite?"*

Ethanol — *"Did you drink alcohol? Did you drink more than usual lately?"*

Sleep Apnea — *"Do you have difficulty sleeping? Do you snore at night? Do you wake up gasping? Are you tired or sleepy during the day?"*

Name / Age

PC - Empathy

SOCRATES—-------------------Impact

Chest pain

CVS Hx - St SoheCo AbviLoC

diet/exercise/stress

DDx **P I R A T E S**

P A M H U G S F O S S

|

S A D

Hypertension

SIGN POST ▶ *"Just to make sure there's nothing serious going on."*

Chest Pain / Headaches / Urinary Changes / *BE FAST / Seizures

▶ C H U D S

"Do you have any chest pain? Any headaches? Any changes in your urine?" BE FAST- *"Did you notice any issues with balance/with your eyes? Any blurring of vision? Any drooping of face, weakness of arm/leg, difficulty swallowing?"* (If all positive, Time to call 911/ go to ER → Alert stroke code)

Any history of seizures? "

Cushing's Syndrome / HyperT /HyperAld / Acromegaly/ CoArctation of Aorta / Pheochromocytoma / Sleep Apnea

C H A P S

SIGN POST DDx: *"I'd like to ask you a few questions to rule out other causes."*

<u>Cushing's Syndrome</u> — *"Have you noticed any weight gain, particularly on your tummy, back of neck and face?"*

Name / Age

PC - Empathy

SOCRATES—-------------------Impact

▶ C H U D S

CVS Hx - St SoheCo AbviLoC

diet/exercise/stress

(↑Salt intake, ↑Lipids, Sedentary Lifestyle)

SIGN POST DDx C H A P S

↱ AM CANDLES

P A M H U G S F O S S

↓ (from P)
-hx of kidney ds
-heart condition
-Endocrine disorder

| (from S) **S A D**

AM CANDLES: (Medications causing HTN - Amphetamine, MAOI, Cocaine, Alcohol, NSAIDs, Decongestants, Lithium, Estrogen/OCP, Steroids)

Hypertension (Continued)

Cushing's Syndrome
HyperT /HyperAld
Acromegaly/ CoArctation of Aorta
Pheochromocytoma
Sleep Apnea

C H A P S

Hyperthyroidism/Hyperaldosteronism — *"Do you feel hot or sweaty when others don't? Have you noticed recent weight loss despite having a good appetite?/ Any muscle weakness?"*

Acromegaly/CoArctation of Aorta — *"Have you noticed any increase in shoe size?/Do you have intermittent pain in your legs? Any lower limb weakness?"*

Pheochromocytoma — *"Any pounding headaches? Have you noticed any palpitations? Any hx of sweating?"*

Sleep Apnea — *"Do you have difficulty sleeping? Do you snore at night? Do you wake up gasping? Are you tired or sleepy during the day?"*

Name / Age

PC - Empathy

SOCRATES—-------------------Impact

C H U D S

CVS Hx - St SoheCo AbviLoC

diet/exercise/stress

(↑Salt intake, ↑Lipids, Sedentary Lifestyle)

SIGN POST DDx C H A P S

↱ AM CANDLES

P A M H U G S F O S S

↓ (from P A M): -hx of kidney ds, -heart condition, -Endocrine disorder

| (from S): **S A D**

AM CANDLES: (Medications causing HTN - Amphetamine, MAOI, Cocaine, Alcohol, NSAIDs, Decongestants, Lithium, Estrogen/OCP, Steroids)

Syncope

(Lightheadedness or fainting)

SOCRATES + Clarify — Was it a seizure or syncope? — *"Did you see any flashy lights before the episode? Were you shaking or having jerky movements? Did you turn blue? Did you bite your tongue? Did you pee yourself? After regaining consciousness, did you notice any numbness or weakness in any part of your body?"*

"Just to make sure there's nothing serious going on."

Glucose, Abuse, Stroke, Panic Attack/Phobia, Stress/Sight, Dehydration, Drugs

G A S P S D d

DDx: *"I'd like to ask you a few questions to rule out other causes."*

Glucose (Hypoglycemia) — *"When was your last meal? Are you hungry? Do you feel shaky? Any hx of eating disorders?"*

Abuse – Ask about social hx, sexual hx and support.

Stroke – N.W.T — *"Any numbness or weakness in any part of your body? Any tingling? Blurry vision? Any hx of heart disease?"*

Name / Age

PC - Empathy

SOCRATES—-------------------Impact

Associated trauma

"Did you hurt yourself at all?"

CVS Hx - St SoheCo AbviLoC

DDx G A S P S D d

P A M H U G S F O S S

|

S A D

Syncope (Continued)

Glucose Abuse Stroke Panic Attack/ Phobia Stress/Sight Dehydration Drugs

G A S P S Dd

<u>Panic Attack/Phobia</u> — *"Are you the kind of person who is anxious a lot? Have you ever had a panic attack? Do you have symptoms of nausea, trembling, chills, choking, sweating, feeling like you might be dying or feeling out of control?"*

<u>Stress/Sight</u> — *"Any recent stressors or emotional news you got recently?/Can you see things well? Any difficulty with vision or hearing?"*

<u>Dehydration (Volume depletion) (Orthostatic hypotension)</u> — *"Any recent hx of diarrhea, vomiting, or blood loss?"* Ask about fluid intake.

<u>Drugs</u> — *"What medications are you taking? Any recent change in dose or addictions of medications?"*

Name / Age

PC - Empathy

SOCRATES——-------------------Impact

Associated trauma

Did you hurt yourself at all?

CVS Hx - St SoheCo AbviLoC

SIGN POST DDx **G A S P S Dd**

P A M   H U G S   F O S S

|

S A D

Congestive Heart Failure (CHF)

Pt comes with SOB on exertion

SOCRATES + **SOB**
– *"Can you walk without symptoms?"*

"Just to make sure there's nothing serious going on."

COPD, Asthma, PE, Pneumonia, Interstitial Lung ds, Arrhythmias (AF,AS)

C A P P I A

DDx *"I'd like to ask you a few questions to rule out other causes."*

<u>COPD</u> — *"Any associated respiratory diseases? Any fever? Do you have a cough? Is it a wet cough?"* If yes, ask **COCA-B**

<u>Asthma</u> — *"Do you have any hx of Asthma? Any allergies? Any whistling or wheezing sound heard when you breathe? Do you use puffers?"*

<u>Pulmonary Embolism</u> — Associated chest pain, worse with breathing (pleuritic pain) "*Have you noticed any pink frothy sputum?*" Ask EAT CHIPS (Refer to PE).

<u>Pneumonia</u> — *"Any hx of fever? Any sick contact or travel history? Any associated cough? Any sputum?"* If yes, ask **COCA-B** <u>Interstitial Lung ds</u> — *"Any hx of lung disease? What is your occupation? Any f/hx of lung diseases?"*

<u>Arrhythmias</u> (Atrial Fib, Aortic Stenosis) – *"Any hx of palpitations or heart racing?"*

Name / Age

PC - Empathy

SOCRATES—-----------------Impact

Chest pain

Dizzy/ faint

CVS Hx - St SoheCo AbviLoC

diet/exercise/stress

DDx C A P P I A

P A M H U G S F O S S

↓ ↪Cialis/Viagra |

Hx of Heart ds
HTN
DM
Cholesterol
Stress

S A D

Deep Vein Thrombosis (DVT)

Pt presents with calf pain/ swelling.

SOCRATES + Ask about associated symptoms → *"Do you have any associated warmth/redness? Did you notice any fever? Did you have a hx of long travel/flight? Any hx of trauma/surgery/immobility? Do you have any associated* ***SOB****? Any chest pain that worsens with breathing (pleuritic pain)? Any hx of cancer? Did you notice any pink frothy sputum?"* For females, ask about pregnancy — *"When was your last menstrual period? Any chance you could be pregnant? Are you on oral contraceptives/hormone replacement therapy/ estrogen?"*

"Just to make sure there's nothing serious going on."

DVT, Cellulitis, PAD, Ankle Sprain/ Achilles Tendinitis, Ruptured Baker's Cyst, Compartment Syndrome, Hematoma

D C P A R C H

DDx: *"I'd like to ask you a few questions to rule out other causes."*

<u>Cellulitis</u> — *"Any local redness/ warmth? Any associate fever?"*

Name / Age

PC - Empathy

SOCRATES------------------------Impact

Chest pain

Loss of consciousness

CVS Hx - St SoheCo AbviLoC

DDx D C P A R C H

P A M H U G S F O S S

|

S A D

Deep Vein Thrombosis (DVT) (Continued)

DVT · Cellulitis · PAD · Ankle Sprain/ Achilles Tendinitis · Ruptured Baker's Cyst · Compartment Syndrome · Hematoma

D C P A R C H

<u>Peripheral artery disease (PAD)</u> — *"Is your leg cold? Is there any associated pain? Do you notice any tingling or numbness? Is your leg paler than the other? Did you notice any weakness or decreased power in the leg?"*

<u>Ankle sprain/ Achilles tendonitis</u> — *"Any history of trauma? Do you feel any tenderness along your ankle or its tendons?"*

<u>Ruptured baker's cyst</u> — *"Was it a sudden onset of pain? Did you have a feeling of fluid down your calf?"*

<u>Compartment syndrome</u> — *"Any trauma? Any numbness, weakness or tingling on your leg? Does the pain worsen with movement?"*

<u>Hematoma</u> — *"hx of Trauma?"*

Name / Age
PC - Empathy

SOCRATES—-------------------Impact

Chest pain

CVS Hx - St SoheCo AbviLoC

SIGN POST DDx **D C P A R C H**

P A M H U G S F O S S

|

S A D

Peripheral Artery Disease (PAD)

SOCRATES + *"Is your leg cold? Is there any associated pain? Do you notice any tingling or numbness? Is your leg paler than the other? Did you notice any weakness or decreased power in the leg?"*

SIGN POST *"Just to make sure there's nothing serious going on."*

DVT, Cellulitis, PAD, Ankle Sprain/ Achilles Tendinitis, Ruptured Baker's Cyst, Compartment Syndrome, Hematoma

D C P A R C H

SIGN POST DDx: *"I'd like to ask you a few questions to rule out other causes."*

<u>DVT</u> — "*Do you have a hx of long travel/flight? Any hx of trauma/surgery/immobility? Do you have any associated SOB? Any chest pain that worsens with breathing (pleuritic pain)? Any hx of cancer? Did you notice any pink frothy sputum?"* For females — *"Are you on oral contraceptives/hormone replacement therapy/ estrogen?"*

<u>Cellulitis</u> — *"Any local redness/ warmth? Any associate fever?"*

<u>Ankle sprain/ Achilles tendonitis</u> — *"Any history of trauma? Do you feel any tenderness along your ankle or its tendons?"*

Name / Age

PC - Empathy

SOCRATES—-------------------Impact

Associated trauma

Chest pain

CVS Hx - St SoheCo AbviLoC

diet/exercise/stress

SIGN POST DDx D C P A R C H

P A M H U G S F O S S

↓ (from P A M): DM, HTN, Hx of Obesity/Weight gain

| (from S): **S A D**

Peripheral Artery Disease (PAD) (Continued)

DVT
Cellulitis
PAD
Ankle Sprain/ Achilles Tendinitis
Ruptured Baker's Cyst
Compartment Syndrome
Hematoma

D C P A R C H

Ruptured baker's cyst — *"Was it a sudden onset of pain? Did you have a feeling of fluid down your calf?"*

Compartment syndrome — *"Any trauma? Any numbness, weakness or tingling on your leg? Does the pain worsen with movement?"*

Hematoma — *"hx of Trauma?"*

Name / Age

PC - Empathy

SOCRATES—-------------------Impact

Associated trauma

Chest pain

CVS Hx - St SoheCo AbviLoC

diet/exercise/stress

DDx D C P A R C H

P A M H U G S F O S S

↓

DM
HTN
Hx of Obesity/Weight gain

S A D

Cough

SOCRATES + Dry cough — *"Any associated sounds? Like a barking sound or a whooping sound with a cough? Have you heard any wheezing or whistling sounds?"*

OR Wet cough – Ask **COCA-B**

"Just to make sure there's nothing serious going on."

Malignancy Asthma GERD Infection CHF

M A G I C

DDx: *"I'd like to ask you a few questions to rule out other causes."*

Malignancy — *"Any weight loss? Night sweats? Fever? Any hx of cancer or f/hx of cancer?"*

Asthma — *"Do you have shortness of breath? Any allergies? Do you use an inhaler? Family hx of asthma?"*

GERD — *"Any chest pain after meals? Any hx of heartburn/sour taste in mouth/chronic cough?"*

Infection (TB/Pneumonia) — *"Do you have a fever? Any hx of sick contacts? Any hx of travel?"*

Congestive Heart Failure — *"Do you have any hx of heart conditions? Any **SOB**?"*

Name / Age

PC - Empathy

SOCRATES——------------------Impact

Constitutional s/s

Weight loss

Fever

CVS Hx - St SoheCo AbviLoC FeTraSic

DDx M A G I C

P A M H U G S F O S S

↓

Ask about occupation/ inhalation of fumes/ insecticides, miners, etc.

Hemoptysis

SOCRATES → Ask **BBL**

"Just to make sure there's nothing serious going on."

Bronchitis Bronchiolitis Aspergillosis TB Tumor Lung Abscess PE Coagulopathy Autoimmune Mitral Stenosis Pneumonia

B A T T L E C A M P

DDx: *"I'd like to ask you a few questions to rule out other causes."*

<u>Bronchitis/ Bronchiolitis</u> — *"Did you have flu-like symptoms such as congestion or sore throat? Have you had a long-standing cough that produces large amounts of sputum?"*

<u>Aspergillosis</u> — *"Do you have a medical condition that has weakened your immune system like a chronic lung disease? Are you on any long-term medications like steroids?"*

<u>Tuberculosis</u> (TB) — *"Have you experienced a persistent cough lasting more than 3 weeks associated with weight loss, night sweats, or fever?" Any hx of sick contacts? Hx of close contact with someone diagnosed with tuberculosis? Any hx of travel?"*

<u>Tumor</u> — *"Any weight loss? Night sweats? Fever? Any hx of cancer or f/hx of cancer?"*

Name / Age

PC - Empathy

SOCRATES——-------------------Impact

Chest pain

Dizzy/ faint

CVS Hx - St SoheCo AbviLoC

DDx **BATTLE CAMP**

P A M H U G S F O S S

|

S A D

Hemoptysis (Continued)

Bronchitis
Bronchiolitis
Aspergillosis
TB
Tumor
Lung Abscess
PE
Coagulopathy
Autoimmune
Mitral Stenosis
Pneumonia

B A T T L E C A M P

Lung Abscess — *"Have you had symptoms like fever, chills or foul-smelling sputum? Or yellow sputum?"*

Pulmonary Embolism (PE) — *"Any chest pain worse with breathing? Any* ***SOB****? Any past hx of DVT?"*

Coagulopathy — *"Do you bruise easily or bleed easily?" Any hx or f/hx of bleeding disorder?"*

Autoimmune — *"Do you have joint pain, skin rashes or red eyes? Do you have a history of an autoimmune disease?"*

Mitral Stenosis — *"Have you ever been told you have a heart murmur? Do you experience shortness of breath with exertion?"*

Pneumonia — *"Are you experiencing chest pain when breathing or shortness of breath? Any fever, chills or yellow sputum?"*

Name / Age

PC - Empathy

SOCRATES—------------------Impact

Chest pain

Dizzy/ faint

CVS Hx - St SoheCo AbviLoC

DDx BATTLE CAMP

P A M   H U G S   F O S S

|

S A D

Asthma

SOCRATES + *"How often has it happened?"*

"Just to make sure there's nothing serious going on."

Infection Medication Outdoor Allergies Indoor Allergies Stress

I M O I S

"I'd like to ask you about a few factors that can be triggers"

Asthma hx — *"When were you diagnosed? Do you use the puffers? How often do you use the puffers? Did you need to increase the intake recently? Did you notice symptoms worsen lately? Any worsening of symptoms during nighttime? How many daytime attacks or worsening of symptoms during daytime? Have you had any ER visits? Ever missed work or activities because of this?"*

Trigger Qs →

Infection — *"Any hx of fever? Any flu-like symptoms? Do you have any red eyes/ runny nose? Ear discharge? Sore throat? Diarrhea/ urinary changes/ joint pain?*

Medication — *"What medications do you take? Any recent changes in dosage? Tell me about your inhalers, are they stored properly? Have you made sure that they aren't expired?"*

Name / Age

PC - Empathy

SOCRATES—-------------------Impact

Chest pain

Dizzy/ faint

CVS Hx - St SoheCo AbviLoC

Triggers I M O I S

P A M H U G S F O S S

|

S A D

Asthma (Continued)

Infection
Medication
Outdoor Allergies
Indoor Allergies
Stress

I M O I S

<u>Outdoor Triggers</u> — *"Do your symptoms occur where it's cold outside/ during exercise? Is it seasonal? Is it due to pollen? Do the symptoms occur when there's smoke/fog/dust/exhaust?"*
<u>Indoor Triggers</u> — *"Does anyone smoke indoors? Do you have any pets? Do you have carpets/thick curtains at home? Do the symptoms get worse when you are around perfume or strong scents? Any construction or renovations at home?"*
<u>Stress</u> — *"Any recent stressors in your life?"*

Name / Age
PC - Empathy

SOCRATES——------------------Impact

Chest pain

Dizzy/ faint

CVS Hx - St SoheCo AbviLoC

Triggers I M O I S

P A M H U G S F O S S

|

S A D

COPD

Patient may complain of chronic cough or SOB

SOCRATES + (Dry cough — *"Any associated sounds? Like a barking sound or a whooping sound with a cough?"*

OR Wet cough – Ask **COCA-B)** + **SOB** - 5 Q's

COPD – (Blue Bloaters) Bronchitis — *"Have you noticed any weight gain? Do you turn blue?"*

(Pink Puffers) Emphysema — *"Have you noticed your skin is pinker? Any hx of repeated chest infections?"*

SIGN POST *"Just to make sure there's nothing serious going on."*

Malignancy Asthma GERD Infection CHF

M A G I C

SIGN POST DDx: *"I'd like to ask you a few questions to rule out other causes."*

Malignancy — *"Any weight loss? Night sweats? Fever? Any hx of cancer or f/hx of cancer?"*

Asthma — *"Do you have shortness of breath? Any allergies? Do you use an inhaler? Family hx of asthma?"*

GERD — *"Any chest pain after meals? Any hx of heartburn/sour taste in mouth/chronic cough?"*

Name / Age

PC - Empathy

SOCRATES——————-Impact

Chest pain

Dizzy/ faint

CVS Hx - St SoheCo AbviLoC FeTraSic

SIGN POST DDx M A G I C

P A M H U G S F O S S

|

S A D

COPD (Continued)

Malignancy Asthma GERD Infection CHF

M A G I C

Infection (TB/Pneumonia) — *"Do you have a fever? Any hx of sick contacts? Any hx of travel?"*

Congestive Heart Failure — *"Do you have any hx of heart conditions? Any **SOB**?"*

Name / Age

PC - Empathy

SOCRATES—------------------Impact

Chest pain

Dizzy/ faint

CVS Hx - St SoheCo AbviLoC FeTraSic

SIGN POST DDx M A G I C

P A M H U G S F O S S

S A D

Pediatrics

How to organise yourself before entering the station + KEY 76
Cough 81
Vomiting 82
Diarrhea - Acute 83
Diarrhea - Chronic 84
Diarrhea - Bloody 85
Constipation 87
Enuresis 89
Hematuria 91
Jaundice 93
Crying Baby 95
Failure to Thrive 97
Delayed Speech 99
Autism 101
Attention Deficit Hyperactivity Disorder (ADHD) 102
Anemia 105
Sudden Infant Death Syndrome (SIDS) 106
Allergy/Anaphylaxis 107
Nephrotic Syndrome 108
Hyperreactive airway Disease 110
Fracture 112
Sleep Disorder 114
Rash 117
Febrile Seizure 119
Obesity 121

How to organise yourself before entering the station

Before entering the station, you will have under two minutes to read the prompt and jot down notes in your booklet.

These notes should focus on key information you'll need to remember while taking the history from the standardized participant (SP). The SP is an actor trained to portray a specific medical condition or scenario. Their purpose is to interact with you and allow the physician examiner (PE) to observe and assess your performance.

The booklet provided is rectangular, about half the size of an A4 sheet. It contains blank sheets for your notes, as well as candidate code stickers, which you'll need to hand over to the examiner before starting each station.

Given the time constraints and anxiety during the station, these notes can serve as a valuable guide to help you complete a thorough history.

Therefore, it is essential to practice responding to prompts and mastering the '2-minute drill' regularly to achieve your best results.

HOW TO PRACTICE :

For practice purposes, folding an A4 sheet in half works well to simulate the booklet.

Hence this book is divided into two columns:

Left column	**Right column**
Contains a breakdown of the mnemonics and the questions you may need to ask.	Notes to write in your booklet as part of your 2-minute drill, often including mnemonics that make the best use of your time and help you recall essential steps efficiently!

These structured notes will provide a clear and concise roadmap to ensure you stay focused and efficient during the station.

The KEY

Knock on the door, Walk in, Wear a smile, Greet the examiner, and hand the candidate code, *"Hi, here's my candidate code."*
Sanitize your hands and simultaneously:

Introduce yourself to the standardized participant (SP):
"Hello, I am Dr___ and I will be your physician today. May I know your name and age, please? How would you like to be addressed? That's great!

"Is it okay if I sit down and take a few notes?"

PC: Presenting Complaints
"What brings you in here today?"
Listen to the patient. It is important to express **Empathy.**
"I am sorry to hear that. That must be quite distressing."

"Okay, so I would like to ask you a few questions and do a physical exam after and we will figure out a treatment plan for you today!"

SOCRATES-B: For conditions with other symptoms SOCRATES-B can still be used.

- site: *"Where is the pain? Can you point at it?"*
- onset: *"Was it gradual or sudden in onset?"*
- character: *"What kind of pain is it? Is it a dull pain or a sharp pain?"*
- radiate: *"Does the pain radiate anywhere?"*
- associated symptoms: *"Any associated symptoms?"*
- time: *"Is the pain constant or intermittent?"*
- exacerbating factor: *"Does anything relieve the pain or make it worse?"*
- severity: *"On a scale from 1-10, how would you rate the pain? 10 being the worst."*
- before: *"Have you had this before?"*

Not every P/C involves pain. Some complaints may just require 'o-ate' onset associated s/s, time, and exacerbating/ relieving factors.

COCA-b: For any vomiting/discharge/sputum/stool/urine.
Colour, **O**dor, **C**onsistency, **A**mount, **B**lood (If yes for blood, ask **BBL**)

BBL — (if pt complains of bleeding), stands for :

- Blood thinners – *"Are you on blood thinners?"*
- Bloody Diarrhea – *"Do you bruise easily or bleed easily?"*
- Liver Disease — *"Any hx of liver disease?"*

Impact: *"How are you coping with this?"*

DDX: Differentials for the condition given for each condition.

SIGNPOST: This symbol means you have to signpost! A signpost is an introductory statement. This is to introduce your segment of questions so the examiner is aware of your line of questioning.

E.g.: DDx - means you have to place an introductory statement before asking for differentials: *"I am going to ask a few questions to rule out any other causes."*

Red flags: This is for conditions we need to rule out right away as they may require urgent attention. **Signpost** — *"Just to rule out anything serious..."*

PAM HUGS FOSS: stands for:

- Past medical hx: *"Since this is the first time we are meeting, do you have any past medical conditions that I should know about? Or that you have been treated for?"*
- Allergies: *"Do you have any allergies?"*
- Medications: *"Are you on any medications? What are the medications? Are you adherent with your medications? What is the dosage?"*
- Hospitalization/Surgery: *"Have you ever had any hospitalization before? Any surgeries done before?"*
- Urinary changes: *"Have you noticed changes in your urine?"*
- GIT changes: *"Have you noticed any changes in your bowel habits?"*
- SAD- **S**moking/**A**lcohol/Recreational **D**rugs:
    - *"Do you smoke? How many cigarettes a day? For how long? Have you ever thought about quitting?"*
    - *"Do you drink alcohol? How often?"*
    - *"Have you done any recreational drugs? What have you used? How do you take it? Do you sniff or inject? Do you share needles?"*
- Family history: *"Any family history of any medical conditions?"* Specific medical conditions you are concerned about.
- Occupation: *"If I may ask, what do you do for a living?"*
- Social: *"May I know about your living conditions? Who do you live with?"*
- Support: *"Do you have any family around? Are they supportive? That's good to know."*

Mnemonics for system questions:
Pediatrics:

FROST DADS

- Fever: *"Any hx of fever?"*
- Rash: *"Any rash on the body?"*
    - If yes, ask **SSSPPP** – Site, Size, Shape, Palpable, Pruritic, Painful.
- Other Organs: Ask for signs of infections in the body. *"Any red eyes? Runny nose? Ear discharge? Neck stiffness? Cough? Abdominal pain? Diarrhea? Urinary issues? Joint Pain? "*
- Swallow: *"Did he swallow anything? Did you notice if he was choking?"*
- Trauma: *"Do you think they hurt themselves?"*
- Diet: *"Are they eating ok?"*
- Activity: *"How is their mood? Are they active? Playful?"*
- Drowsy: *"Have you noticed if your child appears sleepy or drowsy?"*
- Seizures/Sick contacts: *"Have they had any seizures? any sick contacts?"*

Signpost – *"I'd like to ask you a little bit about your child's history starting from the pregnancy, ok?".*

PAD BIN DAF

- Pregnancy – *"How was your pregnancy?/ Did you have a normal pregnancy? Any complications?"*
- Antenatal care – *"Did you have regular follow-up visits? How about your U/S? Was it normal?"*
- Delivery – *"How was the delivery? Any complications?"*
- Birth – *"How was the birth? Was it a Vaginal delivery? Any problems during birth? Do you know the APGAR score?"*
- Immunization – *"Is the immunization up-to-date?"*
- Nutrition – *"How is your child's nutrition? Are they eating well? How is their diet?"*
- Development – *"Is your child touching their milestones on time?"*
- Abuse – *"Are you the primary caregiver? Is your child a happy kid? Is he playful and active? Does he seem to cry a lot? Is anyone around him smoking or drinking? Anyone around him at home seriously ill? Does anyone in the family have mental illness?"*

SOB: Shortness **O**f **B**reath

- *"Is your child able to speak/cry?"*
- *"Do they turn blue?"*
- *"Did you have to take them to the hospital?"*
- *"Do they gasp for air at night?"*
- *"How many pillows do they use?"*

When taking a history with teens:

Confidentiality — *"I would like you to know that everything we talk about will remain between us. I will not be telling your parents or anyone else, ok? However, if it concerns your safety then I will have to tell someone. Ok?"*

HEADSS-

- Home — *"If I may ask about your living conditions, Who do you live with? Are they supportive? Do you have any pets? Do you feel safe at home? Are there any guns or other weapons at home? How are they stored? Do you have access to them?"*
- Education/Employment — *"Do you like your school? How are you fitting in? Do you have friends at school? Do you feel safe at school? Do you face any sort of bullying at all? Do you have a job? What is your workplace environment like?"*
- Activities — *"Do you have any activities you enjoy? Are you in any clubs or teams? Do you drive? Do you exercise? How is your diet?"*
- Drugs (Note: Often teens are more willing to talk about their friends than themselves, so it can be helpful to start with questions about friends.) — *"Do any of your friends' smoke or drink, or do drugs? Have you ever tried? How have you taken it? Did you sniff or inject? Have you ever shared needles? Have you ever been in a car driven by someone who was under the influence or was high on drugs?"*
- Sex – make sure you have asked about confidentiality — *"Are you in a relationship? Are you sexually active? Is it a monogamous relationship? Do you practice safe sex? Have you ever been tested for STIs? Has anyone ever touched you in a way you did not want to be touched or forced you to do something you did not want to do sexually?"*
- Suicidality — *"How has your mood been lately? Have you ever felt low or sad? Have you ever thought about hurting yourself? Have you ever run away from home?"*

Cough

SOCRATES + *"Was it a dry cough or with sputum?"*

If dry — *"Is there a sound with the cough? Like a barking cough or a whooping cough? Any wheeze or whistling heard?"*

If wet — Ask **COCA-b**

"Just to make sure there's nothing serious going on."

Foreign Body, Asthma, GERD, Infection, Cystic Fibrosis

F A G I C

DDx: *"I'd like to ask you a few questions to rule out other causes."*

Foreign Body — *"Do you think they swallowed something? Were they choking?"*

Asthma — *"Does your child have shortness of breath? Any allergies? Does your child use an inhaler? Family hx of asthma?"*

GERD — *"Do they feel fussy after meals? Do they arch their back after meals?"*

Infection — *"Does your child have a fever?"* Ask **FROST DADS.**

Cystic Fibrosis — *"Was your child tested for cystic fibrosis? Did they pass stools after birth? Any repeated infections? Any foul-smelling stools?"*

Name / Age

PC - Empathy

SOCRATES------------------------**Impact**

Is the child toxic

Unable to breathe

Drowsy

Any fever/neck stiffness

F R O S T   D A D S

DDx F A G I C

PEDS Hx - P A D   B I N   D A F

H E A D S S (for teens)

P A M   H U G S

S A D (for teens)

Vomiting

SOCRATES + Ask **COCA-b** (if yes for blood, ask **BBL**)

"Just to make sure there's nothing serious going on."

Pyloric Stenosis
Infection
GERD
Meningitis
Allergies/Abx
TEF

P I G M A T

DDx: *"I'd like to ask you a few questions to rule out other causes."*

Pyloric Stenosis — *"Is it a forceful or projectile vomit especially after feeding? Have you noticed your child still being hungry or wanting to feed again right after vomiting?"*

Infection — Ask **FROST DADS**

GERD — *"Do they feel fussy after meals? Do they arch their back after meals?"*

Meningitis — *"Are they irritable? Have neck stiffness? Do their eyes roll up? Do they have bulging fontanelles?"*

Allergies/Abx — *"Do they have any allergies? Have they taken any antibiotics?"*

Tracheoesophageal Fistula — *"Did you notice your child drooling or choking, especially after feeding? Has your child experienced difficulty swallowing or turning blue while eating?"*

Name / Age

PC - Empathy

SOCRATES——————————Impact

Is the child dizzy/drowsy

Have a high-pitched cry

Any fever/neck stiffness

F R O S T   D A D S

DDx **P I G M A T**

PEDS Hx - P A D   B I N   D A F

H E A D S S (for teens)

P A M   H U G S

S A D (for teens)

Diarrhea - Acute

SOCRATES + Ask **COCA-b**

"Just to make sure there's nothing serious going on."

Sugar (toddler's diarrhea)
Lactose Intolerance
Infection
IBD
Medications
Milk Allergy

s L i i m m

DDx: *"I'd like to ask you a few questions to rule out other causes."*

Sugar (Toddler's diarrhea — *"Does your child drink a lot of sugary drinks?"*
Lactose Intolerance — *"Does your child feel bloated after a feed? Do they pass a lot of gas?"*
Infection — *"Does your child have a fever? Any hx of sick contacts? Any hx of travel? Any intake of street foods recently?"*
Inflammatory Bowel Disease — *"Is there any blood in stools?"* If yes, ask **BBL**. *"Any hx of joint pain? Hx of Red eyes?"*
Medication — *"Is your child taking any medications?"* If yes, ask about dosage/duration.
Milk Allergy — *"Have you noticed your child's symptoms getting worse after consuming milk or dairy products?"*

Name / Age

PC - Empathy

SOCRATES——------------------Impact

Is the child toxic

Dizzy/drowsy

F R O S T D A D S

DDx s L i i m m

PEDS Hx - P A D B I N D A F

H E A D S S (for teens)

P A M H U G S

|

S A D (for teens)

Diarrhea - Chronic

SOCRATES + Ask **COCA-b**

"Just to make sure there's nothing serious going on."

Cystic Fibrosis, Celiac Disease, Constipation, Sugar (toddlers diarrhea), Lactose Intolerance, Infection, IBD, Medications, Milk Allergy

C C C s L i i m m

DDx: *"I'd like to ask you a few questions to rule out other causes."*

Cystic Fibrosis — *"Was your child tested for cystic fibrosis? Did they pass stools after birth? Any repeated infections? Any foul-smelling stools?"*

Celiac Disease — *"Is your child allergic to bread?"*

Constipation — *"Does your child have constipation? How many dirty diapers during the day? Are his stools hard or soft?"*

Sugar (Toddler's diarrhea) — *"Does your child drink a lot of sugary drinks?"*

Lactose Intolerance — *"Does your child feel bloated after a feed? Do they pass a lot of gas?"*

Infection *"Does your child have a fever? Any hx of sick contacts? Any hx of travel? Any intake of street foods recently?"*

Name / Age

PC - Empathy

SOCRATES--------------------Impact

Is the child toxic

Dizzy/drowsy

F R O S T D A D S

DDx CCC sLiimm

PEDS Hx - P A D B I N D A F

H E A D S S (for teens)

P A M H U G S

|

S A D (for teens)

Diarrhea - Bloody

SOCRATES + Ask **COCA-b** (if yes for blood, ask **BBL**)

SIGN POST *"Just to make sure there's nothing serious going on."*

Anal Fissures
Infections/IBD
Rash (HUS/HSP)
Bleeding Disorder
Intestinal Obstruction
Abuse
Trauma

A I R B O A T

SIGN POST DDx: *"I'd like to ask you a few questions to rule out other causes."*

Anal fissures — *"Does your child have pain while passing stools? Have you noticed any streaks of bright red blood on the toilet paper or the surface of stools?"*

Infection (colitis)/ IBD — *"Does your child have a fever? Any hx of sick contacts? Any hx of travel? Any intake of street foods recently? Is there any blood in stools?"* If yes, ask **BBL** *"Any hx of joint pain? Hx of Red eyes?"*

Name / Age

PC - Empathy

SOCRATES—-------------------Impact

Is the child toxic

Dizzy/drowsy

F R O S T D A D S

SIGN POST DDx A I R B O A T

PEDS Hx - P A D B I N D A F

H E A D S S (for teens)

P A M H U G S

|

S A D (for teens)

Diarrhea - Bloody (Continued)

Anal Fissures, Infections/IBD, Rash (HUS/HSP), Bleeding Disorder, Intestinal Obstruction, Abuse, Trauma

A I R B O A T

<u>Rash -Hemolytic Uremic Syndrome (HUS)</u> — *"Has your child developed a rash? Where is the rash?* (Ask **SSSPP**: site/size/ /shape/palpable/pruritic/painful) *Has your child had any episodes of blood in urine? Has your child seemed pale or weak recently? Have they had any unexplained bruising?"*

<u>Henoch Schonlein Purpura (HSP)</u> — *"Has your child complained of any joint pain or swelling recently?"*

<u>Intestinal Obstruction/ Intussusception</u> — *"Does your child have severe abdominal pain where they cry and pull their legs up?"*

<u>Bleeding disorder</u> — *"Does your child bruise easily? Have prolonged bleeding from minor cuts? Do they experience frequent nosebleeds or bleeding gums?"*

<u>Abuse</u> — *"Are you the primary caregiver? Is your child a happy kid? Is he playful and active? Does he seem to cry a lot?"*

<u>Trauma</u> — *"Did your child hurt themselves?"*

Name / Age

PC - Empathy

SOCRATES—------------------Impact

Is the child toxic

Dizzy/drowsy

F R O S T D A D S

SIGN POST DDx **A I R B O A T**

PEDS Hx - P A D B I N D A F

H E A D S S (for teens)

P A M H U G S

S A D (for teens)

Constipation

"Just to make sure there's nothing serious going on."

Diet, Meningomyelocele, imperforate Anus, Thyroid, Cystic Fibrosis, Celiac ds, Hirschsprung ds

d M A T C H

DDx: *"I'd like to ask you a few questions to rule out other causes."*

Diet — *"Can you tell me about their diet? Any changes recently? Water intake? High-fiber diet?"*

Meningomyelocele — *"Does your child have a tuft of hair on their lower back? Any bulge on their lower back?"*

imperforate Anus — *"Did your child pass their stool within the first 1 or 2 days after birth? Have you noticed any abnormality around your child's anal opening?"*

Thyroid —

For Infant — Ask about puffy face, protruding tongue, and bulging fontanelle.

For older children — *"Do they feel cold when others don't?"*

Cystic Fibrosis — *"Was your child tested for cystic fibrosis? Do they have a hx of repeated infections? Did they pass stools at birth?"*

Name / Age

PC - Empathy

SOCRATES—-------------------Impact

Is the child toxic

Dizzy/drowsy

F R O S T D A D S

DDx d M A T C H

PEDS Hx - P A D B I N D A F

H E A D S S (for teens)

P A M H U G S

S A D (for teens)

Constipation (Continued)

Diet — Meningomyelocele — imperforate Anus — Thyroid — Cystic Fibrosis / Celiac ds — Hirschsprung ds

d M A T C H

<u>Celiac Disease</u> — *"Is he allergic to bread?"*

<u>Hirschsprung Disease</u> — *"Did your child pass their stool right after birth? Does he seem bloated after feeding?"*

Name / Age

PC - Empathy

SOCRATES——------------------Impact

Is the child toxic

Dizzy/drowsy

F R O S T D A D S

DDx d M A T C H

PEDS Hx - P A D B I N D A F

H E A D S S (for teens)

P A M H U G S

|

S A D (for teens)

Enuresis

SOCRATES + Ask **COCA-b**

"Just to make sure there's nothing serious going on."

DM/DI, UTI, Neurological Issues, Kidney Stones, Stress, Sleep Apnea, Structural

D U N K S^3

DDx: *"I'd like to ask you a few questions to rule out other causes."*

Diabetes Mellitus/Insipidus — *"Does your child feel thirsty all the time? Does he pee a lot?"*

Neurological Issues – Meningomyelocele — *"Does your child have a tuft of hair on their lower back? Any bulges on their lower back?"*

Urinary Tract infections — *"Does he have a fever? Does your child cry when he pees?"*

Kidney Stones — *"Any hx of kidney disease or kidney stones?"*

Stress — *"Any changes in their life? Is he going to a new school? Any new siblings or additions to your family? Is your child a happy kid? Is he playful and active? Does he seem to cry a lot?"*

Structural — *"Does he have a weak stream or difficulty while peeing?"*

Name / Age

PC - Empathy

SOCRATES——------------------Impact

Is the child toxic

Dizzy/drowsy

F R O S T D A D S

DDx D U N K S^3

PEDS Hx - P A D B I N D A F

H E A D S S (for teens)

P A M H U G S

|

S A D (for teens)

Enuresis (Continued)

DM/DI — UTI — Neurological Issues — Kidney Stones — Stress, Sleep Apnea, Structural

D U N K S^3

<u>Sleep Apnea</u> — *"Does he have difficulty sleeping? Does he snore at night? Does he wake up gasping? Is he tired or sleepy during the day?"*

Name / Age

PC - Empathy

SOCRATES—------------------Impact

Is the child toxic

Dizzy/drowsy

F R O S T D A D S

DDx D U N K S^3

PEDS Hx - P A D B I N D A F

H E A D S S (for teens)

P A M H U G S

S A D (for teens)

Hematuria

SOCRATES + Ask **COCA-b**

"Just to make sure there's nothing serious going on."

Infection Trauma Stones HUS/HSP Exercise Medications Abuse/Alport Syn Tumor Post-Strep GN Diet Ca↑

It's Hemat's DC

DDx: *"I'd like to ask you a few questions to rule out other causes."*

Infection — *"Does he have any fever? Does your child cry when they pee?"*

Trauma — *"Did he hurt themselves?"*

Stones — *"Any hx of kidney disease? Does he complain about severe pain in the lower back or sides? Does it come and go in waves?"*

Hemolytic Uremic Syndrome (HUS) — *"Has your child had any recent episodes of bloody diarrhea? Has your child seemed pale or weak recently? Has he had any unexplained bruising?"*

Henoch Schoenlein Purpura (HSP) — *"Has your child developed a rash? Where is the rash? Has your child complained of any joint pain or swelling recently?"*

Medication — *"Is your child on any medication (e.g. penicillins, analgesics, aminoglycosides, cyclophosphamide)"*

Name / Age

PC - Empathy

SOCRATES——------------------Impact

Is the child toxic

Dizzy/drowsy

Hx of Trauma

F R O S T D A D S

DDx It's Hemat's DC

PEDS Hx - P A D B I N D A F

H E A D S S (for teens)

P A M H U G S

S A D (for teens)

Hematuria (Continued)

Infection, Trauma, Stones, HUS/HSP, Exercise, Medications, Abuse/Alport Syn, Tumor, Post-Strep GN, Diet, Ca↑

It's Hemat's DC

<u>Abuse</u> — *"Is your child a happy kid? Is he playful and active? Does he seem to cry a lot?"*

<u>Alport Syndrome</u> — *"Any hearing loss? Any vision issues? Any family hx of congenital conditions?"*

<u>Tumor</u> — *"Any hx of cancer? Any weight loss? Any lumps or bumps on their body?"*

<u>Post-Strep Glomerulonephritis</u> — *"Has your child had a sore throat in the last few weeks? Any skin infection in the past few weeks?"*

<u>Diet</u> — *"Any change in your child's diet? Does he eat a lot of beetroots? Or blueberries?"*

<u>Hypercalcemia</u> — *"Does he complain of constipation? Muscle weakness? Increased thirst or urination recently?"*

Name / Age

PC - Empathy

SOCRATES--------------------Impact

Is the child toxic

Dizzy/drowsy

Hx of Trauma

F R O S T D A D S

DDx **It's Hemat's DC**

PEDS Hx - P A D B I N D A F

H E A D S S (for teens)

P A M H U G S

S A D (for teens)

Jaundice

"Just to make sure there's nothing serious going on."

Hemolysis, Infection, Trauma, Transfusion Reaction, Thyroid, Galactosemia, BF Jaundice, Biliary Atresia, Polycythemia, Crigler Naijar Syn, CF

H i t t   Ga B Bi   P C C

DDx: *"I'd like to ask you a few questions to rule out other causes."*

<u>Hemolysis</u> (ABO, Rh, Incompatibility) — *"Do you know your baby's blood type group? What is your blood type?"*

<u>Infection</u> — *"Does your child have any fever?"*

<u>Trauma</u> — *"Did your child get hurt at all during the delivery?"*

<u>Transfusion</u> — *"Were they transfused any blood at all?"*

<u>Thyroid</u> — *"Did you notice any puffiness on their face? Notice a large tongue? Do they have difficulty swallowing?"*

<u>Galactosemia</u> —- *"Was your child tested for Galactosemia?"*

<u>Cystic Fibrosis</u> — *"Was your child tested for cystic fibrosis? Do they have a hx of repeated infections? Did they pass stools at birth?"*

Name / Age

PC - Empathy

SOCRATES—------------------Impact

(Ask about encephalopathy)

Is your child drowsy/floppy

Do they have a high-pitched cry

Does your child have weak suckling

F R O S T   D A D S

DDx **Hitt GaBBi PCC**

PEDS Hx - P A D   B I N   D A F

H E A D S S (for teens)

P A M   H U G S

|

S A D (for teens)

Jaundice (Continued)

Hemolysis, Infection, Trauma, Transfusion Reaction, Thyroid, Galactosemia, BF Jaundice, Biliary Atresia, Polycythemia, Crigler Najjar Syn, CF

H i t t Ga B Bi P C C

Breastfeeding Jaundice — *"How many times do you breastfeed your baby? For how long? Does your child seem hungry after a feed? Is your breast still engorged after the feed? Do you give your child formula feed?* (If yes, ask why) *How many wet diapers does your child have in a day? How many dirty diapers? Any change in the urine colour?"*

Polycythemia — *"Does your child have reddish or an overly flushed skin tone?"*

Crigler Najjar Syndrome — Pt may have jaundice that did not respond to phototherapy.

Cystic Fibrosis — *"Was your child tested for cystic fibrosis? Do they have a hx of repeated infections? Did they pass stools at birth?"*

Name / Age

PC - Empathy

SOCRATES—------------------Impact

(Ask about encephalopathy)

Is your child drowsy/floppy

Do they have a high-pitched cry

Does your child have weak suckling

F R O S T D A D S

SIGN POST DDx **Hitt GaBBi PCC**

PEDS Hx - P A D B I N D A F

H E A D S S (for teens)

P A M H U G S

S A D (for teens)

Crying Baby

"Just to make sure there's nothing serious going on."

Colicky Child, Infection, Trauma, Abuse/Neglect, Surgical Condition

C I T A S

DDx: *"I'd like to ask you a few questions to rule out other causes."*

Colicky Child — (Ask duration) *"How often does he cry?* (for > 3 hrs per day for >3 days per week for 3 weeks) *Any chance your child is too hot/ too cold/ needs a diaper change? Have you noticed if there is any diaper rash? Do you burp your child after feeding? Did you try to soothe your child when he cried?"*

Infections — *"Does your child have any fever? Any neck stiffness"*

Trauma — *"Did your child get hurt at all?"*

Abuse / Neglect — *"Do they get hurt often or need to visit the ER frequently? Do they have any bruises on their body? How much time do you spend with them? Does anyone smoke or drink around them? Is there anyone dealing with mental illness around them? Are you the only caregiver? Any other siblings?"*

Name / Age

PC - Empathy

SOCRATES—------------------Impact

Is he floppy/Not responding

Is he turning blue while crying

Any fever/skin rash

Neck stiffness

F R O S T D A D S

DDx C I T A S

PEDS Hx - P A D B I N D A F

H E A D S S (for teens)

P A M H U G S

S A D (for teens)

Crying Baby (Continued)

Colicky Child, Infection, Trauma, Abuse/Neglect, Surgical Condition

C I T A S

Surgical Condition — Needs physical examination to rule out serious conditions such as incarcerated hernia, testicular torsion, anal fissure, calculus or intussusception

Name / Age

PC - Empathy

SOCRATES———————————Impact

Is he floppy/Not responding

Is he turning blue while crying

Any fever/skin rash

Neck stiffness

F R O S T D A D S

DDx C I T A S

PEDS Hx - P A D B I N D A F

H E A D S S (for teens)

P A M H U G S

S A D (for teens)

Failure to Thrive

"Just to make sure there's nothing serious going on."

Diet, Celiac Disease, Lactose Intolerance, DM/DI, UTI, Cystic Fibrosis, hypoThyroid, Abuse, Cardiac ds

d c l d u c t a c

DDx: *"I'd like to ask you a few questions to rule out other causes."*

Diet — *"How's your child's diet? Is he eating well? Did you start giving him/her solid food?"*

Celiac Disease — *"Did you give him/her any bread or cereal? Is he allergic to bread? Did he gain any weight? Do you have his/her growth chart?"*

Lactose Intolerance — *"Does your child feel bloated after a feed? Do they pass a lot of gas? How many dirty diapers?"*

Diabetes Mellitus/Insipidus — *"Does your child feel thirsty all the time? Do they pee a lot?"*

UTI — *"Does he have any fever? Does your child cry when they pee?"*

Cystic Fibrosis — *"Was your child tested for cystic fibrosis? Do they have a hx of repeated infections? Did they pass stools at birth?"*

Hypothyroid — *"Do they feel cold when others don't?"*

Name / Age

PC - Empathy

SOCRATES——------------------Impact

Is he drowsy/ floppy

Do you feel his lips or skin is dry

F R O S T D A D S

DDx **d c l d u c t a c**

PEDS Hx - P A D B I N D A F

H E A D S S (for teens)

P A M H U G S

|

S A D (for teens)

Failure to Thrive (Continued)

Diet, Celiac Disease, Lactose Intolerance, DM/DI, UTI, Cystic Fibrosis, hypoThyroid, Abuse, Cardiac ds

d c l d u c t a c

<u>Abuse</u> — *"Do they get hurt often or need to visit the ER frequently? Do they have any bruises on their body? How much time do you spend with them? Does anyone smoke or drink around them? Is there anyone dealing with mental illness around them? Are you the only caregiver? Any other siblings?"*

<u>Cardiac Disease</u> — *"Any hx of heart disease? Does he have any shortness of breath? Does he turn blue when he cries? Does he wake up gasping for air?"*

Name / Age

PC - Empathy

SOCRATES——------------------Impact

Is he drowsy/ floppy

Do you feel his lips or skin is dry

F R O S T D A D S

SIGN POST DDx d c l d u c t a c

PEDS Hx - P A D B I N D A F

H E A D S S (for teens)

P A M H U G S

S A D (for teens)

Delayed Speech

SOCRATES + *"Did he ever speak at all? How many words? Is he not learning new words?"*

Developmental Delay, Depression, Abuse, Autism, Alcoholic Mom, Structural Abnormality, Hearing Loss, Hypothyroid

D^2 A^3 S H T

DDx: *"I'd like to ask you a few questions to rule out other causes."*

Developmental Delay — Ask about milestones in detail.

Depression — *"Does your child seem more irritable or sad? Does he appear to cry a lot lately?"*

Autism — *"Does he make eye contact? Does he engage people socially? Does he use social gestures while communicating?"*

Abuse — *"Do they get hurt often or need to visit the ER frequently? Do they have any bruises on their body? How much time do you spend with them? Does anyone smoke or drink around them? Is there anyone dealing with mental illness around them? Are you the only caregiver? Any other siblings?"*

Alcoholic Mom — (Fetal Alcohol Syndrome) — *"Did you drink while you were pregnant? How often?"*

Name / Age

PC - Empathy

SOCRATES—-------------------Impact

DDx D^2 A^3 S H T

PEDS Hx - P A D B I N D A F

H E A D S S (for teens)

P A M H U G S

S A D (for teens)

Delayed Speech (Continued)

Developmental Delay, Depression — D^2
Abuse, Autism, Alcoholic Mom — A^3
Structural Abnormality — S
Hearing Loss — H
Hypothyroid — T

D^2 A^3 S H T

Structural Abnormality (e.g. cleft palate) — *"Did you get tested for infections during pregnancy? Any family hx of congenital abnormalities? Does he have difficulty feeding?"*

Hearing Loss — *"Does he have any hearing difficulties or brain infections? Does he respond to you when you call him? Did you notice that he keeps increasing the volume of the TV? Does he get repeated ear infections or brain infections? Did you notice any ear discharge? Was he ever screened for a hearing test when he was born?"*

Hypothyroid — *"Do they feel cold when others don't?"*

Name / Age

PC - Empathy

SOCRATES—-------------------Impact

SIGN POST DDx D^2 A^3 S H T

PEDS Hx - P A D B I N D A F

H E A D S S (for teens)

P A M H U G S

S A D (for teens)

Autism

Patient may come with delayed speech

Developmental Delay, Depression, Abuse, Autism, Alcoholic Mom, Structural Abnormality, Hearing Loss, Hypothyroid

D^2 A^3 S H T

↳ S C R

SIGN POST DDx: *"I'd like to ask you a few questions to rule out other causes."*

Autism (SCR):

- Social Interactions — *"Does he make eye contact? Does he engage people socially? Notice any lack of response to people's emotions?"*
- Communications — *"Does he use speech to express his feelings? Did he ever fantasy play or make-believe play? Does he use any social gestures?"*
- Restricted, Repetitive Behaviour — *"Does he keep a rigid daily schedule? Does he resist any change to it? Does he adapt well to new environments?"*

Ask about possible Risk Factors-

- Infantile Spasms
- Congenital Rubella
- Fragile X syndrome

(Check Delayed Speech for other DDx questions)

Name / Age

PC - Empathy

SOCRATES——-------------------Impact

SIGN POST DDx D^2 A^3 S H T

↳ S C R

PEDS Hx - P A D B I N D A F

H E A D S S (for teens)

P A M H U G S

|

S A D (for teens)

Attention Deficit Hyperactivity Disorder (ADHD)

Δ of ADHD — I - Inattention

H - Hyperactivity

I - Impulsivity

Thyroid, Abuse, Anemia, Drugs, Hearing Loss, other Disorders, Conduct ds, ODD, Autism, Learning Disability, Epilepsy, Depression/ anxiety

T A^2 D H D→coaled

SIGN POST

DDx: *"I'd like to ask you a few questions to rule out other causes."*

ADHD - Inattention — *"Is he easily distracted? Does he have difficulty focusing? Does he jump from one activity to another without finishing it?"*

Hyperactivity — *"Did the teachers complain that your child is full of energy? Does he fidget a lot? Does he refuse to stand still?"*

Impulsivity — *"Is he very impatient? Does he interrupt conversations or other people's activities? Does he talk out of turn?"*

Thyroid — *"Do they feel cold when others don't?"*

Abuse — *"Do they get hurt often or need to visit the ER frequently? Do they have any bruises on their body? How much time do you spend with them? Does anyone smoke or drink around them? Is there anyone dealing with mental illness around them? Are you the only caregiver? Any other siblings?"*

Name / Age

PC - Empathy

SOCRATES---------------------Impact

Δ of ADHD — I - Inattention

H - Hyperactivity

I - Impulsivity

SIGN POST

DDx T A^2DHD→coaled

PEDS Hx - P A D B I N D A F

H E A D S S (for teens)

P A M H U G S

|

S A D (for teens)

Attention Deficit Hyperactivity Disorder (ADHD) (Continued)

Thyroid, Abuse, Anemia, Drugs, Hearing Loss, other Disorders, Conduct ds, ODD, Autism, Learning Disability, Epilepsy, Depression/ anxiety

T A^2 D H D→coaled

<u>Anemia</u> — *"Is he pallor than other kids? Does he get tired easily?"* – Ask about diet, f/hx of bleeding ds, thalassemia, and cancer.

<u>Drugs</u> — *"Is he on any medications?*

<u>Hearing Loss</u> — *"Does he have any hearing difficulties or brain infections? Does he respond to you when you call him? Did you notice that he keeps increasing the volume of the TV? Does he get repeated ear infections or brain infections? Did you notice any ear discharge? Was he ever screened for a hearing test when he was born?"*

<u>Other Disorders:</u>

<u>Conduct disorder</u> – *"Is he aggressive? Does he fight a lot with other kids? Does he like to set fires?"*

<u>Opposition Defiant Disorder</u> – *"Is he resentful; and easily annoyed? Does he argue with adults & is vindictive?"*

<u>Autism</u> – *"Does he make eye contact? Does he have communication skills and can express emotions?"*

<u>Learning Disability</u> – *"Does he like to go to school? Does he have difficulty in reading, writing or mathematics?"*

Name / Age

PC - Empathy

SOCRATES——------------------Impact

Δ of ADHD — I - Inattention

H - Hyperactivity

I - Impulsivity

SIGN POST DDx T A^2DHD→coaled

PEDS Hx - P A D B I N D A F

H E A D S S (for teens)

P A M H U G S

S A D (for teens)

Attention Deficit Hyperactivity Disorder (ADHD) (Continued)

Thyroid, Abuse, Anemia, Drugs, Hearing Loss, other Disorders, Conduct ds, ODD, Autism, Learning Disability, Epilepsy, Depression/ anxiety

T A^2 D H D→coaled

<u>Epilepsy</u> *[Petit-mal Epilepsy] — "Does he have a hx of seizures? Does he have a loss of consciousness, or are there any abnormal movements?"*

<u>Depression/anxiety</u> — *"Has he been stressed recently? Is he anxious or worried a lot? Does he have a past trauma that stressed him a lot? Is he sad? Cries a lot? Does he have nightmares? Is he eating well?"*

Name / Age

PC - Empathy

SOCRATES——------------------Impact

Δ of ADHD — I - Inattention
H - Hyperactivity
I - Impulsivity

SIGN POST DDx T A^2DHD→coaled

PEDS Hx - P A D B I N D A F

H E A D S S (for teens)

P A M H U G S

S A D (for teens)

Anemia

"Just to make sure there's nothing serious going on."

Thalassemia, Anemia of Chronic ds, Iron Deficiency, Lead Poisoning, Sideroblastic, B12 def, Bleeding ds, Bone pain (Tumors)

T A I L S B B B

DDx: *"I'd like to ask you a few questions to rule out other causes."*

Thalassemia — *"Has your child been tested for Thalassemia?"*

Anemia of Chronic Disease — *"Any hx of any past medical condition that your child is being treated for?"*

Iron Deficiency — *"What is your child's diet?"* Ask about the intake of iron-rich food/supplements.

Lead poisoning — *"If you don't mind, I would like to ask about your living conditions. Do you live in a house? Is it an old house or a new renovation?"*

Bleeding Disorders — *"Any hx of bleeding disorders? Does he bruise easily or bleed easily?"*

Bone pain (Tumors/Leukemia) — *"Any hx of weight loss/ fever/ or night sweats? Any lumps or bumps in his body? Any hx of cancer in the family?"*

Name / Age

PC - Empathy

SOCRATES——------------------Impact

Is he drowsy/floppy

Weight loss

Fever

F R O S T D A D S

DDx T A I L S B B B

PEDS Hx - P A D B I N D A F

H E A D S S (for teens)

P A M H U G S

S A D (for teens)

Sudden Infant Death Syndrome (SIDS)

Rule out Risk Factors:

I (Infant Related) M (Mother Related) E (Environment Related)

SIGN POST RF: *"I'd like to ask you a few questions to rule out risk factors."*

<u>Infant Related</u>

- -Prematurity — *"Was your child born on the expected due date?"*
- -Low Birth Weight — *"Do you know what your child's weight was at birth?"*
- -Previous hx of SIDS — *"Any hx of previous siblings who have had unexplained sudden deaths?"*

<u>Mother related</u> — *"Did the mother have regular antenatal visits? Did she drink during pregnancy? Did she smoke? Did she do any drugs during pregnancy?"*

<u>Environment Related</u> — *"Where does your baby sleep? Are there a lot of soft toys in his crib? Does he sleep with anyone other than the caretaker? Does he sleep on his back or his tummy?"*

Name / Age

PC - Empathy

SOCRATES—-------------------Impact

F R O S T D A D S

RF - I M E

PEDS Hx - P A D B I N D A F

H E A D S S (for teens)

P A M H U G S

S A D (for teens)

Allergy/Anaphylaxis

SIGN POST 🚩 *"Just to make sure there's nothing serious going on."*

S/S c c w f a i r s

(Cough, Chest Pain/Tightness, Wheeze, Fever, Allergies, Itching, Rash, Swelling)

F A G I C

(Foreign Body, Asthma, GERD, Infection, Cystic Fibrosis)

SIGN POST DDx: *"I'd like to ask you a few questions to rule out other causes."*

Foreign Body — *"Do you think they swallowed something? Were they choking?"*

Asthma — *"Does your child have shortness of breath? Any allergies? Does your child use an inhaler? Family hx of asthma?"*

GERD — *"Do they feel fussy after meals? Do they arch their back after meals?"*

Infection — *"Does your child have a fever?"* Ask **FROST DADS.**

Cystic Fibrosis — *"Was your child tested for cystic fibrosis? Did they pass stools after birth? Any repeated infections? Any foul-smelling stools?"*

Name / Age

PC - Empathy

SOCRATES———————-Impact

🚩 Difficulty breathing

Turning blue

Loss of consciousness

F R O S T D A D S

Anaphylaxis —> **EpiPen!**

Check Airway, Breathing, Circulation

S/S c c w f a i r s

SIGN POST DDx F A G I C

PEDS Hx - P A D B I N D A F

H E A D S S (for teens)

P A M H U G S

S A D (for teens)

Nephrotic Syndrome

Pt may present with hx of fatigue, swelling of the face, and frothy urine.

SIGN POST *"Just to make sure there's nothing serious going on."*

MCD, Infections, DM, Cystic fibrosis, CHF, Amyloidosis, Plz ask abt Lymphoma, Penicillamine, Kidney

M I D   C A P   failure

SIGN POST DDx: *"I'd like to ask you a few questions to rule out other causes."*

Minimal Change Disease — *"Any hx of kidney disease?"*

Infection – Ask about Malaria, Hepatitis B, and HIV — *"Any hx of travel? Sick contacts?"*

Diabetes Mellitus — *"Does he pee a lot? Is he thirsty a lot?"*

Cystic Fibrosis/Congestive Heart Failure — *"Was your child tested for cystic fibrosis? Do they have a hx of repeated infections? Did they pass stools at birth? Does your child have any hx of heart conditions? Any SOB? Is he able to speak/cry? Does he turn blue? Ever take him to the hospital because of it? Does he gasp during his sleep?"*

Name / Age

PC - Empathy

SOCRATES——————Impact

Is the child toxic

Drowsy

Feeding difficulty

Turning blue

F R O S T   D A D S

SIGN POST DDx **MID CAP failure**

PEDS Hx - P A D   B I N   D A F

H E A D S S (for teens)

P A M   H U G S

|

S A D (for teens)

Nephrotic Syndrome (Continued)

MCD, Infections, DM, Cystic fibrosis, CHF, Amyloidosis, Plz ask abt Lymphoma, Penicillamine, Kidney

M I D C A P failure

SIGN POST DDx: *"I'd like to ask you a few questions to rule out other causes."*

<u>Penicillamine</u> — *"Is your child on any medication?"*

<u>Lymphomas/Tumor</u> – Ask about weight change/pallor/F/hx of cancer

Name / Age

PC - Empathy

SOCRATES——————Impact

Is the child toxic

Drowsy

Feeding difficulty

Turning blue

F R O S T D A D S

SIGN POST DDx **MID CAP failure**

PEDS Hx - P A D B I N D A F

H E A D S S (for teens)

P A M H U G S

S A D (for teens)

Hyperreactive airway Disease

Pt may come with a complaint of cough.

SIGN POST *"Just to make sure there's nothing serious going on."*

Foreign Body, Asthma, GERD, Infection, Cystic Fibrosis

F A G I C

SIGN POST DDx: *"I'd like to ask you a few questions to rule out other causes."* (Check **Cough**)

Infection, Medication, Outdoor Allergies, Indoor Allergies, Stress

Triggers- I M O I S

Infection — *"Any hx of fever? Any flu-like symptoms? Do you have any red eyes/ runny nose? Ear discharge? Sore throat? Diarrhea/ urinary changes/ joint pain?"*

Medication — *"What medications do you take? Any recent changes in dosage? Tell me about your inhalers, are they stored properly? Have you made sure that they aren't expired?"*

Outdoor Triggers — *"Do his symptoms occur where it's cold outside? During exercise? Is it seasonal? Is it due to pollen? Do the symptoms occur when there's smoke/fog/dust/exhaust?"*

Name / Age

PC - Empathy

SOCRATES————————Impact

Difficulty breathing

Turning blue

Loss of consciousness

F R O S T D A D S

Triggers- I M O I S

SIGN POST DDx F A G I C

PEDS Hx - P A D B I N D A F

H E A D S S (for teens)

P A M H U G S

S A D (for teens)

Hyperreactive airway Disease (Continued)

Infection Medication Outdoor Allergies Indoor Allergies Stress

Triggers- I M O I S

<u>Indoor Triggers</u> — *"Does anyone smoke around him? Do you have any pets? Do you have carpets/thick curtains at home? Do his symptoms get worse when he is around perfume or strong scents? Any construction or renovations at home?"*

<u>Stress</u> — *"Any recent stressors in your life?"*

Name / Age

PC - Empathy

SOCRATES————————Impact

Difficulty breathing

Turning blue

Loss of consciousness

F R O S T D A D S

Triggers- I M O I S

DDx F A G I C

PEDS Hx - P A D B I N D A F

H E A D S S (for teens)

P A M H U G S

S A D (for teens)

Fracture

Child with fractures, rule out abuse!

SOCRATES + *"Can you describe what happened? Anyone else get hurt? Any other ER visits before? Do you have other children? Do they have repeated visits to the ER as well?"*

SIGN POST *"Just to make sure there's nothing serious going on."*

Osteogenesis Imperfecta, IBD, Cushing's Syndrome, Ricketts, Abuse, Cystic Fibrosis, Kidney ds, DM, JIA, Thyroid

O! I C R A C K D J T

SIGN POST DDx: *"I'd like to ask you a few questions to rule out other causes."*

<u>Osteopenia Imperfecta</u> — *"Does your child have blue sclera?"*

<u>Inflammatory Bowel Disease</u> — *"Is there any blood in stools? Any hx of joint pain? Hx of Red eyes/mouth ulcers? Does he have complaints of diarrhea? Have you noticed any skin tags around his anal region? Any pain around his anal region?"*

<u>Cushing's Syndrome</u> — *"Did you notice weight gain on his tummy/back of neck/face? Did you notice slow growth in your child?"*

<u>Ricketts</u> — *"Diet? Are his/her teeth falling off?"*

Name / Age

PC - Empathy

SOCRATES——————————Impact

F R O S T D A D S

SIGN POST DDx **O! I CRACKD JT**

PEDS Hx - P A D B I N D A F

H E A D S S (for teens)

P A M H U G S

S A D (for teens)

Fracture (Continued)

Osteogenesis Imperfecta, IBD, Cushing's Syndrome, Ricketts, Abuse, Cystic Fibrosis, Kidney ds, DM, JIA, Thyroid

O! I C R A C K D J T

Abuse / Neglect — *"How much time do you spend with them? Does anyone smoke or drink around them? Is there anyone dealing with mental illness around them? Are you the only caregiver? Any other siblings?"*

Signs of Neglect – Immunization is not on time or up to date, there is a delay in seeking medical attention, inadequate food intake, inadequate supervision, poor weight gain, and decreased time spent with the child. *"How many hours do you spend with him? Is he a difficult child?"*

Cystic Fibrosis — *"Was your child tested for cystic fibrosis? Do they have a hx of repeated infections? Did they pass stools at birth?"*

Kidney Disease — *"Any hx of kidney disease?"*

Diabetes Mellitus — *"Does he pee a lot? Is he thirsty a lot?"*

Juvenile Idiopathic Arthritis — *"Any hx of joint pain/joint swelling?"*

"Hyperthyroidism — *"Does your child feel hot when others don't?"*

Name / Age

PC - Empathy

SOCRATES————————Impact

F R O S T D A D S

DDx **O! I CRACKD JT**

PEDS Hx - P A D B I N D A F

H E A D S S (for teens)

P A M H U G S

S A D (for teens)

Sleep Disorder

Ask questions about sleep hygiene in the order of BEFORE, DURING, AFTER.

BEFORE: *"Is there a bedtime routine, like wearing PJ's, brushing teeth, tucking in bed? Does he eat before sleeping/heavy meals/late meals? Any sugary drinks before bedtime? Do you read in bed? Does he watch a screen or iPad in bed? Does he sleep in a dark or lit room?"*

DURING: *"Does he wake up during the night? How often? Does he snore? Did you notice him gasp for air while sleeping? Does he make any jerky movts? Did he complain of nightmares? Does he wake up screaming from his sleep? Do you find it hard to console him at that time? Does he wet the bed? Did you notice him walk around during his sleep/perform tasks while sleeping?"*

AFTER: *"Does he feel unrefreshed or tired when he wakes up? Does he complain of any morning headaches? Did he ever mention hallucinations while drifting into sleep or drifting out of it? Did he ever collapse suddenly when excited or surprised?"*

Sleep Apnea, Anxiety, Asthma, Autism, ADHD, Abuse, Growing Pains, Parasomnias, Depression, Drugs

sl a a a a a p p D d

Name / Age

PC - Empathy

SOCRATES——————————Impact

Ask questions about sleep hygiene (before/during/after)

SIGN POST DDx slaaaaapp D d

PEDS Hx - P A D B I N D A F

H E A D S S (for teens)

P A M H U G S

|

S A D (for teens)

Sleep Disorder (Continued)

Sleep Apnea, Anxiety, Asthma, Autism, ADHD, Abuse, Growing Pains, Parasomnias, Depression, Drugs

sl a a a a a p p D d

Sleep Apnea — *"Do they have difficulty sleeping? Do they snore at night? Do they wake up gasping? Are they tired or sleepy during the day?"*

Anxiety — *"Is he anxious? Does he worry a lot? Any new stressors in his life? Any bullying at school?"*

Asthma — *"Does your child have shortness of breath? Any allergies? Does your child use an inhaler? Family hx of asthma?"*

Autism — *"Does he make eye contact? Does he engage people socially? Does he use any social gestures?"*

ADHD (Ask IHI)

- Inattention — *"Is he easily distracted? Does he have difficulty focusing? Does he jump from one activity to another without finishing it?"*
- Hyperactivity — *"Did the teachers complain that your child is full of energy? Does he fidget a lot? Does he refuse to stand still?"*
- Impulsivity — *"Is he very impatient? Does he interrupt conversations or other people's activities? Does he talk out of turn?"*

Name / Age

PC - Empathy

SOCRATES————————Impact

Ask questions about sleep hygiene (before/during/after)

SIGN POST DDx **slaaaaapp D d**

PEDS Hx - P A D B I N D A F

H E A D S S (for teens)

P A M H U G S

S A D (for teens)

Sleep Disorder (Continued)

Sleep Apnea, Anxiety, Asthma, Autism, ADHD, Abuse, Growing Pains, Parasomnias, Depression, Drugs

sl a a a a a p p D d

<u>Abuse</u> — *"Does he get hurt often and need to visit the ER a lot? Does he have any bruises on his body? How much time do you spend with your child? Does anyone smoke or drink around him? Is anyone dealing with a mental illness around him? Have you ever had to speak to Child Aid Society in the past?"*

<u>Growing Pains</u> — *"Does he complain of leg pain and wake up at night because of it?"*

<u>Parasomnias</u> — *"Have you noticed him sleepwalking? Does he complain about nightmares? Night terrors? Any hx of Narcolepsy?"*

<u>Depression</u> — *"Is he focused on schoolwork? How are his grades? Is he irritable? Does he cry a lot? How's his appetite? Any weight changes?"*

<u>Drugs</u> — *"Is he on any medications/steroids/antidepressants?"*

Name / Age

PC - Empathy

SOCRATES——————————Impact

Ask questions about sleep hygiene (before/during/after)

SIGN POST DDx **slaaaaapp D d**

PEDS Hx - P A D B I N D A F

H E A D S S (for teens)

P A M H U G S

S A D (for teens)

Rash

SOCRATES + SSS PPP + Ask **COCA-b** if there is discharge.

Two types of Rash: Blanchable & Non-blanchable

"Just to make sure there's nothing serious going on."

Meningococcal Meningitis, Abuse, HUS, HSP, ITP

M a h h i

DDx: *"I'd like to ask you a few questions to rule out other causes."*

Meningococcal Meningitis — *"Does he have a fever? Neck stiffness?"*

Abuse — *"Does he get hurt often and need to visit the ER a lot? Does he have any bruises on his body? How much time do you spend with your child? Does anyone smoke or drink around him? Is anyone dealing with a mental illness around him> Have you ever had to speak to Child Aid Society in the past?"*

Hemolytic Uremic Syndrome (HUS) — *"Does your child have hx of bloody diarrhea? Does he seem paler than others? Have you noticed easy bruising on your child? Any changes in urine?"*

Name / Age

PC - Empathy

SOCRATES——------------------Impact

+ SSS PPP: (Site, Size, Shape, Palpable, Pruritus, Painful)

Does he have a fever

Neck stiffness

Drowsy/floppy

F R O S T D A D S

DDx **M a h h i**

PEDS Hx - P A D B I N D A F

H E A D S S (for teens)

P A M H U G S

S A D (for teens)

Rash (Continued)

Meningococcal Meningitis — Abuse — HUS — HSP — ITP

M a h h i

Henoch Schonlein Purpura (HSP) —

"Where is the rash? Has your child complained of any joint pain or swelling recently?"

Immune Thrombocytopenia Purpura —

"Any hx of flu-like symptoms before? Any fever? Any hx of bleeding from nose, gums or elsewhere?"

Name / Age

PC - Empathy

SOCRATES———————————Impact

\+ SSS PPP: (Site, Size, Shape, Palpable, Pruritus, Painful)

Does he have a fever

Neck stiffness

Drowsy/floppy

F R O S T D A D S

SIGN POST

DDx **M a h h i**

PEDS Hx - P A D B I N D A F

H E A D S S (for teens)

P A M H U G S

|

S A D (for teens)

Febrile Seizure

Take a detailed history of the seizure:

BEFORE: *"Any trauma? Any hx of seizures before? Is your child on any medications?"*
DURING: *"Did your child hurt themselves? Did he bite his tongue? Did he pee himself? Was his whole body shaking, or only part of his body? How long did it last?"*
AFTER: *"How was he doing after? Was he able to respond to you? Did he have any weaknesses in any part of his body?"*

Ask **FROST DADS**

Fever, Infection, Tumor, Sleep/ Stress, Trauma, Epilepsy, Electrolytes, Drugs

F i t s T e e d

SIGN POST DDx: *"I'd like to ask you a few questions to rule out other causes."*

<u>Infection</u> — *"Does he have any fever? Does your child cry when they pee?"*
<u>Tumor</u> — *"Any hx of cancer? Any weight loss? Any lumps or bumps on their body?*
<u>Sleep/Stress</u> — *"Any difficulty sleeping or sleep disorders? Any recent stressors in your life?"*
<u>Trauma</u> — *"Did they hurt themselves?" rule out abuse."*

Name / Age

PC - Empathy

SOCRATES—-------------------Impact

Any fever

Neck stiffness

Drowsy/floppy

F R O S T D A D S

SIGN POST DDx **F i t s T e e d**

PEDS Hx - P A D B I N D A F

H E A D S S (for teens)

P A M H U G S

S A D (for teens)

Febrile Seizure (Continued)

Fever, Infection, Tumor, Sleep/ Stress, Trauma, Epilepsy, Electrolytes, Drugs

F i t s T e e d

<u>Epilepsy</u> *[Petit-mal Epilepsy] — "Have you noticed your child suddenly stop what they are doing and stare blankly for a few seconds and then resume activity immediately after? Do these episodes occur frequently throughout the day without warning?"*

<u>Electrolytes</u> — *"How often does he breastfeed?/ (older child – "How is his diet etc.?") Is he dehydrated? Sunken eyes? Dry lips?"*

<u>Drugs</u> — *"Is he on any medications?"*

Name / Age

PC - Empathy

SOCRATES—-------------------Impact

Any fever

Neck stiffness

Drowsy/floppy

F R O S T D A D S

DDx **F i t s T e e d**

PEDS Hx - P A D B I N D A F

H E A D S S (for teens)

P A M H U G S

S A D (for teens)

Obesity

Inform about confidentiality.

Diet — *"I'd like to know about your diet. What do you have for breakfast/lunch/dinner? How many snacks?"*

Activities — *"Do you do any physical activities? Any physical activities you enjoy doing? How much screen time do you get in a day?"*

Rule out Eating disorders — *"How long has the weight been a concern? Do you think your weight is ideal or more than ideal? Has the weight gain been slow over time or sudden? Do you ever throw up after eating food? Do you hide what you eat from others or eat in secret?"*

Rule out PCOS, Thyroid disease ,Cushing syndrome, Carpenter Syndrome, Turner syndrome.

Name / Age

PC - Empathy

SOCRATES—------------------Impact

🚩 F/hx of DM, Heart disease, high cholesterol

F R O S T   D A D S

PEDS Hx - P A D   B I N   D A F

H E A D S S (for teens)

P A M   H U G S

|

S A D (for teens)

Musculoskeletal System

How to organise yourself before entering the station + KEY 123

Single Joint Pain 128

Multiple Joint Pain 130

Rheumatoid Arthritis 132

Gout 133

Neck Pain 134

Shoulder Pain 136

Carpal Tunnel Syndrome 138

Hip Pain 139

Knee Pain 141

Acute Back Pain 144

Chronic Back Pain 146

Ankle Pain 149

Fatigue 151

How to organise yourself before entering the station

Before entering the station, you will have under two minutes to read the prompt and jot down notes in your booklet.

These notes should focus on key information you'll need to remember while taking the history from the standardized participant (SP). The SP is an actor trained to portray a specific medical condition or scenario. Their purpose is to interact with you and allow the physician examiner (PE) to observe and assess your performance.

The booklet provided is rectangular, about half the size of an A4 sheet. It contains blank sheets for your notes, as well as candidate code stickers, which you'll need to hand over to the examiner before starting each station.

Given the time constraints and anxiety during the station, these notes can serve as a valuable guide to help you complete a thorough history.

Therefore, it is essential to practice responding to prompts and mastering the '2-minute drill' regularly to achieve your best results.

HOW TO PRACTICE:

For practice purposes, folding an A4 sheet in half works well to simulate the booklet.

Hence this book is divided into two columns:

Left column	**Right column**
Contains a breakdown of the mnemonics and the questions you may need to ask.	Notes to write in your booklet as part of your 2-minute drill, often including mnemonics that make the best use of your time and help you recall essential steps efficiently!

These structured notes will provide a clear and concise roadmap to ensure you stay focused and efficient during the station.

The KEY

Knock on the door, Walk in, Wear a smile, Greet the examiner, and hand the candidate code, *"Hi, here's my candidate code."*
Sanitize your hands and simultaneously:

Introduce yourself to the standardized participant (SP):
"Hello, I am Dr___ and I will be your physician today. May I know your name and age, please? How would you like to be addressed? That's great!

"Is it okay if I sit down and take a few notes?"

PC: Presenting Complaints
"What brings you in here today?"
Listen to the patient. It is important to express **Empathy.**
"I am sorry to hear that. That must be quite distressing."

"Okay, so I would like to ask you a few questions and do a physical exam after and we will figure out a treatment plan for you today!"

SOCRATES-B: For conditions with other symptoms SOCRATES-B can still be used.

- site: *"Where is the pain? Can you point at it?"*
- onset: *"Was it gradual or sudden in onset?"*
- character: *"What kind of pain is it? Is it a dull pain or a sharp pain?"*
- radiate: *"Does the pain radiate anywhere?"*
- associated symptoms: *"Any associated symptoms?"*
- time: *"Is the pain constant or intermittent?"*
- exacerbating factor: *"Does anything relieve the pain or make it worse?"*
- severity: *"On a scale from 1-10, how would you rate the pain? 10 being the worst."*
- before: *"Have you had this before?"*

Not every P/C involves pain. Some complaints may just require 'o-ate' onset associated s/s, time, and exacerbating/ relieving factors.

COCA-b: For any vomiting/discharge/sputum/stool/urine.
Colour, **O**dor, **C**onsistency, **A**mount, **B**lood (If yes for blood, ask **BBL**)

BBL — (if pt complains of bleeding), stands for :

- Blood thinners – *"Are you on blood thinners?"*
- Bloody Diarrhea – *"Do you bruise easily or bleed easily?"*
- Liver Disease — *"Any hx of liver disease?"*

Impact: *"How are you coping with this?"*

DDX: Differentials for the condition given for each condition.

SIGN POST **SIGNPOST:** This symbol means you have to signpost! A signpost is an introductory statement. This is to introduce your segment of questions so the examiner is aware of your line of questioning.

E.g.: SIGN POST DDx - means you have to place an introductory statement before asking for differentials: *"I am going to ask a few questions to rule out any other causes."*

Red flags: This is for conditions we need to rule out right away as they may require urgent attention.

PAM HUGS FOSS: stands for:

- Past medical hx: *"Since this is the first time we are meeting, do you have any past medical conditions that I should know about? Or that you have been treated for?"*
- Allergies: *"Do you have any allergies?"*
- Medications: *"Are you on any medications? What are the medications? Are you adherent with your medications? What is the dosage?"*
- Hospitalization/Surgery: *"Have you ever had any hospitalization before? Any surgeries done before?"*
- Urinary changes: *"Have you noticed changes in your urine?"*
- GIT changes: *"Have you noticed any changes in your bowel habits?"*
- SAD- **S**moking/**A**lcohol/Recreational **D**rugs:
  - *"Do you smoke? How many cigarettes a day? For how long? Have you ever thought about quitting?"*
  - *"Do you drink alcohol? How often?"*
  - *"Have you done any recreational drugs? What have you used? How do you take it? Do you sniff or inject? Do you share needles?"*
- Family history: *"Any family history of any medical conditions?"* Specific medical conditions you are concerned about.
- Occupation: *"If I may ask, what do you do for a living?"*
- Social: *"May I know about your living conditions? Who do you live with?"*
- Support: *"Do you have any family around? Are they supportive? That's good to know."*

Mnemonics for system questions:
Musculoskeletal System:

Rheumatology hx taking — **NIFTI**

- Neuro (NWT b/b) — *"Any numbness/ weakness/ tingling? Any changes in your bowel habits? Any urinary changes? Have you ever had an accident regarding your bowel habits? If I may ask, do you feel it when you wipe?"* (asking for saddle anesthesia)
- Infection (Fever, UTIs, Pneumonia) — Ask about fever, and urinary changes (↑Frequency, urgency, any associated burning) Ask about IVDU, travel hx, sexual hx, STIs, tattoos, piercing and discharge.
- Fracture/Trauma (Ask about tetanus immunization) — *"Did you hurt yourself? Did you do any heavy lifting lately?"* Ask about occupation/ work hazards. If MVA (motor vehicle accident) ask about other passengers/ helmets/ seatbelts/ Tetanus shots.
- Tumor (Constitutional s/s, family hx of CA) — "Any hx of cancer? Any weight loss? Any lumps or bumps on their body?
- Inflammation (mnemonic **Mr. Round)**
  - Morning Stiffness — *"Do you have Morning Stiffness?"*
  - Red Eyes — *"Any Red Eyes?"*
  - Rashes — *"Have you noticed any Rashes on your face/body?"*
  - Other — *"Any Other joint pain?"*
  - Ulcers — *"Have you noticed any Ulcers? Mouth Ulcers or genital Ulcers?"*
  - Nail changes — *"Any Nail changes?"*
  - Diarrhea — *"Any Diarrhea or abdominal pain?"*

FOR SYSTEMIC LUPUS ERYTHEMATOSUS (SLE) - **MD SOAP PHEN**

- Malar Rash — *"Do you have a rash on your face?"*
- Discoid Rash — *"Do you have a discord rash on your body?"*
- Skin changes — *"Have you noticed pallor skin/ have you noticed that your skin is pale as compared to others?"(anemia)*
- Oral Ulcers — *"Have you noticed any ulcers in your mouth?"*
- Arthritis/ Anemia — *"Do you experience joint pain?"*
- Proteinuria/ Photosensitivity — *"Have you noticed a sensitivity to light?"*
- Pancreatitis —*"Any yellowing of the skin? Any frothy urine or greasy stools?"*
- Hepatitis — *"Have you noticed any yellowing of the skin?"*
- Eye Changes — *"Any red eyes?"*
- Neurological Changes — *"Any headaches? Seizures?"*

FOR ANKYLOSING SPONDYLITIS (AS) - **BUN FACED PA**

- Back Pain
- Uveitis
- N - Good response to NSAIDS
- F/x of AS
- Arthritis
- Crohn's Disease
- Enthesitis
- Dactylitis
- Psoriasis
- Aortic Regurgitation (Ask about exercise tolerance, SOB, and chest pain)

Single Joint Pain

"Just to make sure there's nothing serious going on."

OA SA Tumor RA Infection Crystal A. Hemarthrosis (Trauma)

O S T R I C H

DDx: *"I'd like to ask you a few questions to rule out other causes."*

Osteoarthritis (OA) — *"Do you experience any morning stiffness? How long does it last? Is the joint pain relieved by rest/ worse at the end of the day? Other joints involved?"*

Septic Arthritis (SA) — *"Is the joint pain associated with redness/ swelling? warmth/ fever? Any hx of previous infections? Any hx of UTIs? Burning micturition? H/x of IVDU?"*

Tumor — *"Any hx of cancer? Any family hx of cancer? Any weight loss? Any lumps or bumps on their body? Any fever/ night sweats?"*

Rheumatoid Arthritis (RA) — Morning stiffness lasts ↑ ½ hour, Symmetrical joint pain relieved by activity. Can ask about any nodules on fingers.

Infection — Ask about fever, s/s of UTIs, and other infections e.g. pneumonia, pericarditis, meningitis, or previous hx of infection.

Name / Age

PC - Empathy

SOCRATES——------------------Impact

Trauma

Septic arthritis (fever, warmth, swelling, redness)

DDx **O S T R I C H**

N I F T I hx

P A M H U G S F O S S

S A D

Single Joint Pain (Continued)

OA SA Tumor RA Infection Crystal A. Hemarthrosis (Trauma)

O S T R I C H

Crystal Arthropathies (Gout/Pseudogout) — Associated with sudden onset of pain (usually big toe) with redness, swelling, and warmth. *"Has this ever happened before? Any nodules or lesions on your ears?"* Ask about diet/ medication/ alcohol/ meat/ seafood/ dehydration.

Hemarthrosis/ Trauma — *"Did you hurt yourself? Any h/x of bleeding disorders? Blood thinners?"* Ask about Tetanus immunization.

Name / Age

PC - Empathy

SOCRATES——————————Impact

Trauma

Septic arthritis (fever, warmth, swelling, redness)

SIGN POST DDx O S T R I C H

N I F T I hx

P A M   H U G S   F O S S

S A D

Multiple Joint Pain

SIGN POST *"Just to make sure there's nothing serious going on."*

Gout RA OA Sjogren Syn SLE PsA EA AS ReA

G R O S S P E A R

SIGN POST DDx: *"I'd like to ask you a few questions to rule out other causes."*

Gout — Associated with sudden onset of pain (usually big toe) with redness, swelling and warmth. *"Has this ever happened before? Any nodules or lesions on your ears?"* Ask about diet/ medication/ alcohol/ meat/ seafood/ dehydration.

Rheumatoid Arthritis (RA) — Morning stiffness lasts ↑ ½ hour. Symmetrical joint pain relieved by activity. Can ask about any nodules on fingers.

Osteoarthritis (OA) — *"Do you experience any morning stiffness? How long does it last? Is the joint pain relieved by rest/ more at the end of the day? Other joints involved?"*

Sjogren Syndrome — *"Have you noticed dry eyes? For how long? (usually ↑ 3 months) Do you notice any sand-like sensation in your eyes? Do you use artificial tears? Have you noticed dry mouth? Do you drink a lot of water while eating?"*

Name / Age

PC - Empathy

SOCRATES—-------------------**Impact**

Trauma

Septic arthritis (fever, warmth, swelling, redness)

SIGN POST DDx **G R O S S P E A R**

N I F T I hx

P A M H U G S F O S S

|

S A D

Multiple Joint Pain (Continued)

Gout RA OA Sjogren Syn SLE PsA EA AS ReA

G R O S S PEAR

Systemic Lupus Erythematosus (SLE) — *"Have you noticed any rashes on your face or body? Have you experienced sensitivity to light? Have you noticed that your skin is paler than others? Have you had any oral ulcers? Any weakness/ fatigue/ fever?"*

Also, check Key – **MD SOAP PHEN**

Psoriatic Arthritis (PsA) — *"Have you noticed any red, scaly rashes on your body? Any nail changes/pitting on nails? Any joint pain in your fingers?"*

Enteropathic Arthritis (EA) — *"Any hx of diarrhea before the joint pain? Hx of Crohn's disease or ulcerative colitis?"*

Ankylosing Spondylitis (AS) — *"Do you experience back pain? How long?* (↑3 months) *Is it relieved by medications like Ibuprofen? Do you have red eyes? Nail changes?"*

Reactive Arthritis (ReA) — *"Do you have any urinary changes? Burning micturition? Any d/c? Fever? Any red eyes?"*

Name / Age

PC - Empathy

SOCRATES---------------------**Impact**

Trauma

Septic arthritis (fever, warmth, swelling, redness)

SIGN POST DDx G R O S S P E A R

N I F T I hx

P A M H U G S F O S S

S A D

Rheumatoid Arthritis

SIGN POST 🚩 *"Just to make sure there's nothing serious going on."*

Gout	RA	OA	Sjogren Syn	SLE	PsA	EA	AS	ReA
G	R	O	S	S	P	E	A	R

SIGN POST DDx: *"I'd like to ask you a few questions to rule out other causes."*
(Check MULTIPLE JOINT PAIN)

A little info on RA:

Poor Prognostic Factors:

20	Y	E	E	R
↑ 20 Jts	Young Age	↑ESR	Extra Articular Features	↑Risk Factors

Extra Articular Features:

S	C	R	E	E	N	L	B
Skin Changes	Cardiac	Renal	Eye	Endocrine	Neuro	Lung	Blood

Skin Changes — Rheumatoid Nodules/ Palpable Purpura

Cardiac — Myocarditis/ Valvular disease

Renal — Amyloidosis

Eye — Keratoconjunctivitis

Endocrine — Hashimoto's Thyroiditis

Neuro – Peripheral Neuropathy

Lung — Fibrosis/ Effusion/ Inflammatory Nodules

Blood — (Felty's Syndrome) Splenomegaly + Neutropenia

Name / Age

PC - Empathy

SOCRATES—-------------------**Impact**

🚩 Trauma

Septic arthritis (fever, warmth, swelling, redness)

SIGN POST DDx GROSS PEAR

Ask RA Questions

- Pt will have symmetrical joint pain, especially on the fingers.
- Morning stiffness ↑ 1 hour, worse with rest, better with activity.
- Pt may have fatigue, myalgia, and depression.
- Ask about finger deformity/ ulnar deviation.
- 🚩 RF → Smoking

N I F T I hx

P A M H U G S F O S S

S A D (from S of HUGS)

Gout

SIGN POST "*Just to make sure there's nothing serious going on.*"

OA SA Tumor RA Infection Crystal A. Hemarthrosis (Trauma)

O S T R I C H

SIGN POST DDx: *"I'd like to ask you a few questions to rule out other causes."* *(Check SINGLE JOINT PAIN)*

Gout Qs

- *"Any nodules or lesions on your ears?*
- *Any hx of Kidney Stones?"* (↑ Uric Acid)
- Diet: S A L T
  - Seafood Alcohol Liver/Turkey (Red Meat)
- Medications: F A C T P E
  - Furosemide
  - Aspirin
  - Cyclophosphamide
  - Thiazide Diuretics
  - Pyrazinamide
  - Ethambutol

Name / Age

PC - Empathy

SOCRATES——-------------------**Impact**

Trauma

Septic arthritis (fever, warmth, swelling, redness)

SIGN POST DDx O S T R I C H

Ask Gout Qs

- Sudden onset of pain associated with swelling/ redness/ warmth → goes away in 5-10 days.
- May have prior hx of similar symptoms. *"Has this ever happened to you before?"*
- Ask about diet/ medication/ atrophy/ kidney stones.

N I F T I hx

P A M H U G S F O S S

S A D

Neck Pain

SIGN POST 🚩 *"Just to make sure there's nothing serious going on."*

CR CM Infection Trauma RA OA Depression
R M I T R O D

SIGN POST DDx: *"I'd like to ask you a few questions to rule out other causes."*

Cervical Radiculopathy (CR) — *"Any shooting and/or burning pain? Does it radiate down your shoulders? Any numbness, weakness or tingling?"*

Cervical Myelopathy (CM) — *"Any gait disturbances/difficulty walking? Any muscle wasting/ muscle cramps? b/b - any bowel or bladder changes?"*

Infection — *"Any fever? Neck stiffness/ nausea & vomiting? Any local warmth/ redness/swelling?"*

Trauma — *"Did you hurt yourself?"* Ask about Tetanus immunization.

Rheumatoid Arthritis (RA) — Morning stiffness lasts ↑ ½ hour. Symmetrical joint pain relieved by activity. Can ask about any nodules on fingers.

Osteoarthritis (OA) — *"Do you experience any morning stiffness? How long does it last? Is the joint pain relieved by rest?/ worse at the end of the day? Other joints involved?"*

Name / Age

PC - Empathy

SOCRATES—-------------------**Impact**

🚩 Rule out trauma/ whiplash injury

Septic arthritis (fever, warmth, swelling, redness)

SIGN POST DDx **R M I T R O D**

N I F T I hx

P A M H U G S F O S S

S A D

Neck Pain (Continued)

CR CM Infection Trauma RA OA Depression

R M I T R O D

<u>Depression</u> — *"How has your mood been lately? Are you feeling depressed / decreased concentration/feelings of guilt? Have you thought of hurting yourself?"*

Name / Age

PC - Empathy

SOCRATES———————————**Impact**

Rule out trauma/ whiplash injury

Septic arthritis (fever, warmth, swelling, redness)

SIGN POST DDx **R M I T R O D**

N I F T I hx

P A M H U G S F O S S

S A D

Shoulder Pain

SIGN POST 🚩 *"Just to make sure there's nothing serious going on."*

Rotator Cuff, Adhesive Capsulitis, Slap Tendonitis, Arthritis, CR, PMR, Trauma, DMM

R A S A C P T D

SIGN POST DDx: *"I'd like to ask you a few questions to rule out other causes."*

<u>Rotator Cuff tear/impingement</u> — *"Do you experience weakness in your arm? Loss of arm movement? Pain on lifting arms above your heads? Pain on sleeping on that side?"*

<u>Adhesive Capsulitis</u> — Gradual onset, limited active and passive movements, worse at night. Pt may be an older female with DM, hx of trauma, immobilization, stroke, MI, or hypothyroidism. *"Have you ever been experiencing limited movement of your arm?"*

<u>Slap Tendonitis</u> — O'Brien's test positive.

<u>Arthritis</u> (SA, RA, OA) — *"Do you experience any morning stiffness? Is the joint pain relieved by rest? Is joint pain more at the end of the day? Other joints involved? Is the joint pain associated with any redness/ swelling/ fever?"* Can ask about nodules on fingers.

Name / Age

PC - Empathy

SOCRATES——-------------------**Impact**

🚩 Trauma

Septic arthritis (fever, warmth, swelling, redness)

SIGN POST DDx **R A S A C P T D**

N I F T I hx

P A M H U G S F O S S

|

S A D

Shoulder Pain (Continued)

Rotator Cuff, Adhesive Capsulitis, Slap Tendonitis, Arthritis, CR, PMR, Trauma, DMM

R A S A C P T D

<u>Cervical Radiculopathy</u> — *"Any shooting and/or burning pain? Does it radiate down your shoulders? Any numbness, weakness or tingling?"*

<u>Polymyalgia Rheumatica</u> (PMR) — *"Do you have pain/ stiffness on both shoulders? Do you notice this more in the morning? Is this associated with fatigue?/ fever?/ weight loss? Do you have difficulty putting on a shirt?"*

<u>Trauma</u> — *"Did you hurt yourself?"* Ask about Tetanus immunization.

<u>Dermatomyositis (DMM)</u> — *"Do you have trouble combing your hair/ getting up from a chair/ lifting heavy objects? Have you noticed any purple rashes on your eyelids or your knuckles? Have you noticed that you are tired most of the time? Any difficulty swallowing? Any hx of cancer or family hx of cancer?"*

Name / Age

PC - Empathy

SOCRATES---------------------**Impact**

Trauma

Septic arthritis (fever, warmth, swelling, redness)

SIGN POST DDx **R A S A C P T D**

N I F T I hx

P A M H U G S F O S S

S A D

Carpal Tunnel Syndrome

Pt complaints of wrist pain, worse at night.

SIGN POST *"Just to make sure there's nothing serious going on."*

OA, SA, Tumor, RA, Infection, Crystal A., Hemarthrosis (Trauma)

O S T R I C H

SIGN POST DDx: *"I'd like to ask you a few questions to rule out other causes."*

(Check SINGLE JOINT PAIN)

<u>CTS Qs-</u>

- Ask abt pain at night/ NWT (numbness, weakness, tingling sensation) and occupation.
- Associated with RA, DM, Hypothyroidism, Acromegaly

Name / Age

PC - Empathy

SOCRATES—-------------------**Impact**

Trauma

Septic arthritis (fever, warmth, swelling, redness)

SIGN POST DDx O S T R I C H

N I F T I hx

P A M H U G S F O S S

|

S A D

Hip Pain

SIGN POST 🚩 *"Just to make sure there's nothing serious going on."*

AS Gout RA OA OM PsA EA ReA FAI Tumor Referred Pain

A GROOPER FTR

SIGN POST DDx: *"I'd like to ask you a few questions to rule out other causes."*

Ankylosing Spondylitis (AS) — *"Do you experience back pain? How long?* (↑3 months) *Is it relieved by medications like Ibuprofen? Have you noticed any red eyes? Any nail changes?"*

Gout — Associated with sudden onset of pain (usually big toe) with redness, swelling and warmth. *"Has this ever happened before? Any nodules or lesions on your ears?"* Ask about diet/ medication/ alcohol/ meat/ seafood/ dehydration.

Rheumatoid Arthritis (RA) — Morning stiffness lasts ↑ ½ hour. Symmetrical joint pain relieved by activity. Can ask about any nodules on fingers.

Osteoarthritis (OA) — *"Do you experience any morning stiffness? How long does it last? Is the joint pain relieved by rest/ more at the end of the day? Other joints involved?"*

Name / Age

PC - Empathy

SOCRATES———————————-**Impact**

🚩 Trauma

Septic arthritis (fever, warmth, swelling, redness)

SIGN POST DDx **A GROOPER FTR**

N I F T I hx

P A M H U G S F O S S

S A D

Hip Pain (Continued)

AS Gout RA OA OM PsA EA ReA FAI Tumor Referred Pain

A G R O O P E R F T R

Osteomyelitis (OM) — *"Is the joint pain associated with any fever/redness/ swelling? warmth? Any hx of previous infections? Any hx of UTIs? Burning micturition/ chest pain/ palpitations/ neck stiffness/shortness of breath?"*

Psoriatic Arthritis (PsA) — *"Have you noticed any red scaly rashes on your body? Any nail changes/pitting on nails? Any joint pain in your fingers?"*

Enteropathic Arthritis (EA) — *"Any hx of diarrhea before the joint pain? Hx of Crohn's disease or ulcerative colitis?"*

Reactive Arthritis (ReA) — *"Do you have any urinary changes? Burning micturition? Any d/c? Fever? Any red eyes?"*

Femoral Acetabular Impingement (FAI) – Pt will have pain/ stiffness. May develop a limp. Pt avoids activities that increase the pain — *"Does it hurt when you tie a shoelace, ride a bike or sit for too long?"*

Tumor — *"Any hx of cancer? Any family hx of cancer? Any weight loss? Any lumps or bumps on their body? Any fever/ night sweats?"*

Referred Pain — Can be due to kidney stone, pyelonephritis, pancreas, abdominal aortic aneurysm etc.

Name / Age

PC - Empathy

SOCRATES—------------------**Impact**

Trauma

Septic arthritis (fever, warmth, swelling, redness)

SIGN POST DDx A GROOPER FTR

N I F T I hx

P A M H U G S F O S S

S A D

Knee Pain

"Just to make sure there's nothing serious going on."

Sprain, Patellofemoral Syn, Osgood Schlatter, Referred pain, Trauma/Tumor
Gout, RA, OA / OM, Osteoporosis, PsA, EA, ReA

SPORT GROOPER

DDx: *"I'd like to ask you a few questions to rule out other causes."*

Sprain/Ligament tear — *"Did you hurt yourself? Do you play any sports? Any pain when you use the stairs? Do you hear any audible pop in your knees when you turn?"*

Patellofemoral Syndrome — *"Do you notice knee pain when you squat or sit for too long?"*

Osgood Schlatter – Teen with a painful lump on the tibial tuberosity. Pain when jumping or kneeling. Relieved by rest. Differentiate from growing pains — *"How is your sleep?"*

Trauma — *"Did you hurt yourself?"*

Tumor — *"Any hx of cancer? Any family hx of cancer? Any weight loss? Any lumps or bumps on their body? Any fever/ night sweats?"*

Name / Age

PC - Empathy

SOCRATES——------------------**Impact**

Trauma

Septic arthritis (fever, warmth, swelling, redness)

DDx **SPORT GROOPER**

NIFTI hx

P A M H U G S F O S S

S A D

Knee Pain (Continued)

Sprain, Patellofemoral Syn, Osgood Schlatter, Referred pain, Trauma/Tumor

S P O R T

Gout, RA, OA / OM, Osteoporosis, PsA, EA, ReA

GROOPER

Gout — Associated with sudden onset of pain (usually big toe) with redness, swelling, and warmth. *"Has this ever happened before? Any nodules or lesions on your ears?"* Ask about diet/ medication/ alcohol/ meat/ seafood/ dehydration.

Rheumatoid Arthritis (RA) — Morning stiffness lasts ↑ ½ hour. Symmetrical joint pain relieved by activity. Can ask about any nodules on fingers.

Osteoarthritis (OA) — *"Do you experience any morning stiffness? How long does it last? Is the joint pain relieved by rest?/ more at the end of the day? Other joints involved?"*

Osteomyelitis (OM) — *"Is the joint pain associated with any fever/redness/ swelling? warmth? Any hx of previous infections? Any hx of UTIs? Burning micturition/ chest pain/ palpitations/ neck stiffness/shortness of breath?"*

Osteoporosis — Any h/x of falls? Hx of previous f#? Ask about menopause and medications.

Name / Age

PC - Empathy

SOCRATES—-------------------**Impact**

Trauma

Septic arthritis (fever, warmth, swelling, redness)

DDx **SPORT GROOPER**

N I F T I hx

P A M H U G S F O S S

|

S A D

Knee Pain (Continued)

Sprain, Patellofemoral Syn, Osgood Schlatter, Referred pain, Trauma/Tumor

S P O R T

Gout, RA, OA / OM, Osteoporosis, PsA, EA, ReA

GROOPER

<u>Psoriatic Arthritis</u> (PsA) — *"Have you noticed any red scaly rashes on your body? Any nail changes/pitting on nails? Any joint pain in your fingers?"*

<u>Enteropathic Arthritis</u> (EA) — *"Any hx of diarrhea before the joint pain? Hx of Crohn's disease or ulcerative colitis?"*

<u>Reactive Arthritis</u> (ReA) — *"Do you have any urinary changes? Burning micturition? Any d/c? Fever? Any red eyes?"*

Name / Age

PC - Empathy

SOCRATES--------------------**Impact**

Trauma

Septic arthritis (fever, warmth, swelling, redness)

SIGN POST DDx**SPORT GROOPER**

N I F T I hx

P A M H U G S F O S S

|

S A D

Acute Back Pain

SOCRATES + *"Relieved by any particular position? (Standing, sitting, bending forward or backwards).*

"Just to make sure there's nothing serious going on."

Spasm, Spondylolisthesis, Trauma, OM / HZ, Sciatica, disc Herniation, FAI, Referred Pain

S T O S H F R

DDx: *"I'd like to ask you a few questions to rule out other causes."*

<u>Spondylolisthesis</u> — Lower back pain radiates to the buttocks, ↑ with activity or trauma, relieved by sitting or change in position (Neurogenic Claudication)

<u>Spasm/Trauma</u> — *"Did you hurt yourself? Have you been lifting anything heavy?"*

<u>Osteomyelitis (OM)/ Herpes Zoster</u> — *"Is the pain associated with any local redness/ swelling/ warmth/ fever/ rashes or lesions? Any hx of previous infections? Any hx of UTIs? Burning micturition? palpitations? neck stiffness?"*

<u>Sciatica</u> — Sharp, shooting pain. Radiates down the leg or buttocks.

<u>Disc Herniation</u> — NWT (numbness, weakness, tingling) Sharp shooting pain.

Name / Age

PC - Empathy

SOCRATES——-------------------**Impact**

Acute onset

b/b (Bowel/ Bladder changes)

Saddle anesthesia (Rule out cauda equina syndrome)

Trauma

Septic arthritis (fever, warmth, swelling, redness)

DDx **S T O S H F R**

N I F T I hx

P A M H U G S F O S S

S A D

Acute Back Pain (Continued)

Spasm, Spondylolisthesis — S
Trauma — T
OM / HZ — O
Sciatica — S
disc Herniation — H
FAI — F
Referred Pain — R

S T O S H F R

Femoral Acetabular Impingement (FAI) – Pt will have pain/ stiffness. May develop a limp. Pt avoids activities that increase the pain — *"Does it hurt when you tie a shoelace, ride a bike or sit for too long?"*

Referred Pain — Can be due to kidney stones, pyelonephritis, pancreas, AAA (abdominal aortic aneurysm) etc.

Name / Age

PC - Empathy

SOCRATES——------------------**Impact**

Acute onset

b/b (Bowel/ Bladder changes)

Saddle anesthesia (Rule out cauda equina syndrome)

Trauma

Septic arthritis (fever, warmth, swelling, redness)

SIGN POST DDx: S T O S H F R

N I F T I hx

P A M H U G S F O S S

S A D

Chronic Back Pain

SIGN POST 🚩 *"Just to make sure there's nothing serious going on."*

Mechanical Back Pain, OA, OP, OM, PsA, EA, AS, RA, SLE / Sjogren's Syn, Spondylosis, Spinal Stenosis, Tumor

MOOO Pear SSST

SIGN POST DDx: *"I'd like to ask you a few questions to rule out other causes."*

Mechanical Back Pain — *"Do you have any hx of recent injury, heavy lifting or any activity that could have strained your back muscles?"*

Osteoarthritis (OA) — *"Do you experience any morning stiffness? How long does it last? Is the joint pain relieved by rest? worse at the end of the day? Other joints involved?"*

Osteoporosis — *"Any h/x of falls? Hx of previous f#?"* Ask about menopause and medications.

Osteomyelitis (OM) — *"Is the joint pain associated with any fever/redness/ swelling? warmth? Any hx of previous infections? Any hx of UTIs? Burning micturition/ palpitations/ neck stiffness?"*

Name / Age

PC - Empathy

SOCRATES—-------------------Impact

🚩 TUNA FISH

T - Tumor / Trauma

U - Unintentional weight loss

N - Neurological Signs (b/b NWT)

A - Age ↑50 yrs

F - Fever

I - IV Drug User (IVDU)

S - Steroid use

H - Hx of Cancer

Signs of septic arthritis

SIGN POST DDx

MOOO Pear SSST

N I F T I hx

P A M H U G S F O S S

S A D

Chronic Back Pain (Continued)

Mechanical Back Pain, OA, OP, OM, PsA, EA, AS, RA, SLE / Sjogren's Syn, Spondylosis, Spinal Stenosis, Tumor

MOOO Pear SSST

<u>Psoriatic Arthritis</u> (PsA) — *"Have you noticed any red, scaly rashes on your body? Any nail changes/pitting on nails? Any joint pain in your fingers?*

<u>Enteropathic Arthritis</u> (EA) — *"Any hx of diarrhea before the joint pain? Hx of Crohn's disease or ulcerative colitis?"*

<u>Reactive Arthritis</u> (ReA) — *"Do you have any urinary changes? Burning micturition? Any d/c? Fever? Any red eyes?"*

<u>Ankylosing Spondylitis</u> (AS) — *"Do you experience back pain? How long? (↑3* months) *Is it relieved by medications like Ibuprofen? Have you noticed any red eyes? Any nail changes?"*

<u>Rheumatoid Arthritis</u> (RA) — Morning stiffness lasts ↑ ½ hour. Symmetrical joint pain relieved by activity. Can ask about any nodules on fingers.

<u>Systemic Lupus Erythematosus</u> (SLE) — *"Have you noticed any rashes on your face or body? Have you experienced sensitivity to light? Have you noticed that your skin is paler than others? Have you had any oral ulcers? Any weakness/ fatigue/ fever?"*

MD SOAP PHEN

Name / Age

PC - Empathy

SOCRATES————————Impact

T U N A F I S H

T - Tumor / Trauma

U - Unintentional weight loss

N - Neurological Signs (b/b NWT)

A - Age ↑50 yrs

F - Fever

I - IV Drug User (IVDU)

S - Steroid use

H - Hx of Cancer

Signs of septic arthritis

DDx

MOOO Pear SSST

N I F T I hx

P A M   H U G S   F O S S

S A D

Chronic Back Pain (Continued)

Mechanical Back Pain, OA, OP, OM, PsA, EA, AS, RA, SLE / Sjogren's Syn, Spondylosis, Spinal Stenosis, Tumor

MOOO Pear SSST

<u>Spinal Stenosis</u> — Pain relieved by bending forward like pushing a trolley, increases on bending backwards like climbing stairs (Kemp's sign).

<u>Spondylosis</u> — Seen in chronic back abusers (i.e. Gymnasts, weightlifters, backpackers, labourers. Ask about activities/occupation.)

<u>Tumor</u> — *"Any hx of cancer? Any family hx of cancer? Any weight loss? Any lumps or bumps on their body? Any fever/ night sweats?"*

Name / Age

PC - Empathy

SOCRATES—------------------Impact

TUNA FISH

T - Tumor / Trauma

U - Unintentional weight loss

N - Neurological Signs (b/b NWT)

A - Age ↑50 yrs

F - Fever

I - IV Drug User (IVDU)

S - Steroid use

H - Hx of Cancer

Signs of septic arthritis

SIGN POST DDx

MOOO Pear SSST

N I F T I hx

P A M H U G S F O S S

S A D

Ankle Pain

"Just to make sure there's nothing serious going on."

Gout OA AT Trauma PF Arthritis Cellulitis Tarsal Tunnel Syn Bunion

GOAT PACT B

DDx: *"I'd like to ask you a few questions to rule out other causes."*

Crystal Arthropathies (Gout/Pseudogout) — Associated with sudden onset of pain (usually big toe) with redness, swelling, and warmth. *"Has this ever happened before? Any nodules or lesions on your ears?"* Ask about diet/ medication/ alcohol/ meat/ seafood/ dehydration.

Osteoarthritis (OA) — *"Do you experience any morning stiffness? How long does it last? Is the joint pain relieved by rest?/worse at the end of the day? Other joints involved?"*

Achilles Tendonitis — *"I'd like to know if you wear shoes that fit well. Do you wear heels often? Did you notice burning/ swelling/ stiffness in your ankle?"*

Trauma — *"Did you hurt yourself/ had a fall? Do you play any sports? (Squash, tennis, basketball) Did the pain start during the game? Did you hear a pop sound? Do you ever get steroid injections? Are you on any medications? (e.g. fluoroquinolones)"*

Name / Age

PC - Empathy

SOCRATES———————Impact

Trauma- (sprain/ tendon rupture/ dislocation/ fracture /compartment syndrome)

Signs of Septic Arthritis

DDx GOAT PACT B

N I F T I hx

P A M   H U G S   F O S S

S A D

Ankle Pain (Continued)

Gout OA AT Trauma PF Arthritis Cellulitis Tarsal Tunnel Syn Bunion

G O A T P A C T B

<u>Plantar fasciitis (PF)</u> — Ask about activity/ occupation (*runner/ athlete/dancer*). *"Is there morning stiffness? Do you have pain when walking from rest? Does it increase at the end of the day or with prolonged standing? Do you have pain when you point your toes upward?* (Toe Dorsiflexion)*"*

<u>Arthritis</u> — Ask questions about septic arthritis/ other joints/ associated red eyes, skin changes/ UTIs.

<u>Cellulitis</u> — *"Is the pain associated with any skin redness/ warmth or swelling? Do you have a fever?"*

<u>Tarsal Tunnel Syndrome</u> (Due to tibial nerve entrapment) — *"Did you have any numbness, burning, or tingling in your heel, arch of your foot, or your toes? Have you noticed any difficulty in moving your toes?"*

<u>Bunion</u> (pain in toe/foot) — *"Have you noticed any visible bumps at the base of your big toe? Any pain/ swelling around the big toe when wearing shoes? Has your big toe started to lean towards the other toe?"*

Name / Age

PC - Empathy

SOCRATES—-------------------Impact

Trauma- (sprain/ tendon rupture/ dislocation/ fracture /compartment syndrome)

Signs of Septic Arthritis

SIGN POST DDx **GOAT PACT B**

N I F T I hx

P A M H U G S F O S S

S A D

Fatigue

PMR DMM MG Thyroid Cushing's Steroids Statins SLE RA

PD My T C S S SR

DDx: *"I'd like to ask you a few questions to rule out other causes."*

Polymyalgia Rheumatica (PMR) — *"Do you have pain/ stiffness in both shoulders? Do you notice this more in the morning? Is this associated with fatigue/ fever/ weight loss? Do you have difficulty putting on a shirt?"*

Dermatomyositis (DMM) — *"Do you have trouble combing your hair/ getting up from a chair/ lifting heavy objects? Have you noticed any purple rashes on your eyelids or your knuckles? Have you noticed that you are tired most of the time? Any difficulty swallowing? Any hx of cancer or family hx of cancer?"*

Myasthenia gravis — *"Do you notice any tiredness at the end of day? Any drooping of eyelids end of day?"*

Thyroid — Ask about celiac disease, hx of gastrectomy or intestinal resection, and IBD.

Name / Age

PC - Empathy

SOCRATES———————-Impact

DDx **PD My TCSS SR**

N I F T I hx

P A M H U G S F O S S

S A D

Fatigue (Continued)

PMR DMM MG Thyroid Cushing's Steroids Statins SLE RA

PD My T C S S SR

<u>Cushing's Syndrome</u> — *"Have you noticed any weight gain, particularly on your tummy, back of neck, and face?"*

<u>Hypothyroidism</u> — *"Do they feel cold when others don't?"*

<u>Medications</u> — *"Are you on medications like Steroids? Statins?"* Ask about dosage and duration.

<u>Systemic Lupus Erythematosus</u> (SLE) — *"Have you noticed any rashes on your face or body? Have you experienced sensitivity to light? Have you noticed that your skin is paler than others? Have you had any oral ulcers? Any weakness/ fatigue/ fever?"*

MD SOAP PHEN

<u>Rheumatoid Arthritis</u> (RA) — Morning stiffness lasts ↑ ½ hour. Symmetrical joint pain relieved by activity. Can ask about any nodules on fingers.

Name / Age

PC - Empathy

SOCRATES—-------------------Impact

SIGN POST DDx **PD My TCSS SR**

N I F T I hx

P A M H U G S F O S S

S A D

Gastrointestinal System

How to organise yourself before entering the station + KEY **154**

Hematemesis/ Melena **158**

Acute Diarrhea **160**

Chronic Diarrhea **161**

Bloody Diarrhea **163**

Acute Abdominal Pain **165**

Abdominal Pain — Elderly **1667**

Chronic Abdominal Pain **168**

Bright Red Blood Per rectum (BRBPR) **170**

Dysphagia **172**

Jaundice **175**

How to organise yourself before entering the station

Before entering the station, you will have under <u>two minutes</u> to read the prompt and jot down notes in your booklet.

These notes should focus on key information you'll need to remember while taking the history from the standardized participant (SP). The SP is an actor trained to portray a specific medical condition or scenario. Their purpose is to interact with you and allow the physician examiner (PE) to observe and assess your performance.

The booklet provided is rectangular, about half the size of an A4 sheet. It contains blank sheets for your notes, as well as candidate code stickers, which you'll need to hand over to the examiner before starting each station.

Given the time constraints and anxiety during the station, these notes can serve as a valuable guide to help you complete a thorough history.

Therefore, it is essential to practice responding to prompts and mastering the '2-minute drill' regularly to achieve your best results.

HOW TO PRACTICE :

For practice purposes, folding an A4 sheet in half works well to simulate the booklet.

Hence this book is divided into two columns:

Left column	**Right column**
Contains a breakdown of the mnemonics and the questions you may need to ask.	Notes to write in your booklet as part of your <u>2-minute drill</u>, often including mnemonics that make the best use of your time and help you recall essential steps efficiently!

These structured notes will provide a clear and concise roadmap to ensure you stay focused and efficient during the station.

The KEY

Knock on the door, Walk in, Wear a smile, Greet the examiner, and hand the candidate code, "*Hi, here's my candidate code.*"
Sanitize your hands and simultaneously:

Introduce yourself to the standardized participant (SP):
"*Hello, I am Dr___ and I will be your physician today. May I know your name and age, please? How would you like to be addressed? That's great!*

"*Is it okay if I sit down and take a few notes?*"

PC: Presenting Complaints
"*What brings you in here today?*"
Listen to the patient. It is important to express **Empathy.**
"*I am sorry to hear that. That must be quite distressing.*"

"*Okay, so I would like to ask you a few questions and do a physical exam after, and we will figure out a treatment plan for you today!*"

SOCRATES-B: For conditions with other symptoms, SOCRATES-B can still be used.

- site: "*Where is the pain? Can you point at it?*"
- onset: "*Was it gradual or sudden in onset?*"
- character: "*What kind of pain is it? Is it a dull pain or a sharp pain?*"
- radiate: "*Does the pain radiate anywhere?*"
- associated symptoms: "*Any associated symptoms?*"
- time: "*Is the pain constant or intermittent?*"
- exacerbating factor: "*Does anything relieve the pain or make it worse?*"
- severity: "*On a scale from 1-10, how would you rate the pain? 10 being the worst.*"
- before: "*Have you had this before?*"

Not every P/C involves pain. Some complaints may just require 'o-ate' onset associated s/s, time, and exacerbating/ relieving factors.

COCA-b: For any vomiting/discharge/sputum/stool/urine.
Colour, **O**dor, **C**onsistency, **A**mount, **B**lood (If yes for blood, ask **BBL**)

BBL — (if pt complains of bleeding), stands for :

- Blood thinners – "*Are you on blood thinners?*"
- Bloody Diarrhea – "*Do you bruise easily or bleed easily?*"
- Liver Disease — "*Any hx of liver disease?*"

Impact: "*How are you coping with this?*"

DDX: Differentials for the condition given for each condition.

SIGNPOST: This symbol means you have to signpost! A signpost is an introductory statement. This is to introduce your segment of questions so the examiner is aware of your line of questioning.

E.g.: DDx - means you have to place an introductory statement before asking for differentials: *"I am going to ask a few questions to rule out any other causes."*

Red flags: This is for conditions we need to rule out right away as they may require urgent attention.

PAM HUGS FOSS: stands for:

- Past medical hx: *"Since this is the first time we are meeting, do you have any past medical conditions that I should know about? Or that you have been treated for?"*
- Allergies: *"Do you have any allergies?"*
- Medications: *"Are you on any medications? What are the medications? Are you adherent with your medications? What is the dosage?"*
- Hospitalization/Surgery: *"Have you ever been hospitalized before? Any surgeries done before?"*
- Urinary changes: *"Have you noticed changes in your urine?"*
- GIT changes: *"Have you noticed any changes in your bowel habits?"*
- SAD- **S**moking/**A**lcohol/Recreational **D**rugs:
  - *"Do you smoke? How many cigarettes a day? For how long? Have you ever thought about quitting?"*
  - *"Do you drink alcohol? How often?"*
  - *"Have you done any recreational drugs? What have you used? How do you take it? Do you sniff or inject? Do you share needles?"*
- Family history: *"Any family history of any medical conditions?"* Specific medical conditions you are concerned about.
- Occupation: *"If I may ask, what do you do for a living?"*
- Social: *"May I know about your living conditions? Who do you live with?"*
- Support: *"Do you have any family around? Are they supportive? That's good to know."*

Mnemonics for system questions:
GIT History Taking:

PaN V BHT GaSY
P - Abdominal Pain
Nausea
Vomiting, if yes, ask **COCA-b**

BHT GaSY
Bloating — *"Are you experiencing any bloating?"*
Heartburn
Travel hx
Gas — *"Are you able to pass gas?"*
Swallowing difficulty —
Yellow Skin

Hematemesis/ Melena

Pt complains of coffee coloured vomiting/ or black tarry stools

SOCRATES + **COCA-b** → ask **BBL**

"Just to make sure there's nothing serious going on."

Ulcers, Varices, AVM, Mallory Weiss / Borhave Syn, Esophagitis, Cancer

U V A M E C

DDx: *"I'd like to ask you a few questions to rule out other causes."*

Ulcers:

- Gastric ulcer — *"Do you experience any chest pain after eating? Heartburn? Sour taste in your mouth? Hx of smoking?"*
- Duodenal ulcer — *"Do you have any tummy pain that is relieved by eating?"*
- Stress ulcer — *"Any recent stressors? ICU/ Hospital visits? Any anxiety?"*
- NSAIDS — *"Have you been taking any medication for pain? Any Ibuprofen?"*

Varices — *"Any hx of liver disease? Any change in skin colour? yellowing of the skin? pale stools? Dark urine? itchiness? increase in abdominal girth?"*

Name / Age

PC - Empathy

SOCRATES——------------------Impact

Stable/ Faint

SOB

Anemia/ Fatigue

Ask **BBL**:

- Blood thinners – *"Are you on blood thinners?"*
- Blood disorders – *"Do you bruise easily or bleed easily?"*
- Liver Disease — *"Any hx of liver disease?"*

DDx U V A M E C

GIT Hx - Pan v BHT GaSY

P A M H U G S F O S S

|

S A D

Hematemesis/ Melena (Continued)

Ulcers — U
Varices — V
AVM — A
Mallory Weiss / Borhave Syn — M
Esophagitis — E
Cancer — C

U V A M E C

<u>Mallory Weiss/ Boerhaave Syndrome</u> — *"Did you have forceful projectile vomiting?"*

<u>Esophagitis</u> — *"Have you experienced painful swallowing?"* Ask if pt is immunocompromised. *"Do you have DM? Are you on any steroids? Immunosuppressants? Have you been tested for HIV?"* May also ask about IV drug use/ sexual hx.

<u>Cancer</u> — *"Any history of weight loss, fever, or night sweats? Any hx of cancer or family hx of cancer?"*

Name / Age

PC - Empathy

SOCRATES——------------------Impact

Stable/ Faint

SOB

Anemia/ Fatigue

Ask **BBL**:

- Blood thinners – *"Are you on blood thinners?"*
- Blood disorders – *"Do you bruise easily or bleed easily?"*
- Liver Disease — *"Any hx of liver disease?"*

DDx U V A M E C

GIT Hx - Pan v BHT GaSY

P A M H U G S F O S S

|

S A D

Acute Diarrhea

SOCRATES + **COCA-b** → yes? Ask **BBL**

"Just to make sure there's nothing serious going on."

Stressors, Lactose Intolerance, Infections, IBD, Meds, Thyroid

S L i i M T

DDx: *"I'd like to ask you a few questions to rule out other causes."*

<u>Stressors</u> — *"Any recent stressors or any emotional news you've gotten recently?"*

<u>Lactose Intolerance</u> — *"Are you lactose intolerant? Do you feel bloated or pass a lot of gas after consuming milk or dairy products?"*

<u>Infection</u> — *"Do you have a fever? Any hx of sick contacts? Any hx of travel? Any intake of street foods recently?"*

<u>Inflammatory Bowel Disease</u> (IBD) — *"Is there any blood in the stools?"* If yes, ask **BBL**. *"Any hx of joint pain? Hx of red eyes?"*

<u>Medications</u> – Abx/ Allergy meds — *"Are you taking any medications?" If yes,* ask about dosage/duration.

<u>Thyroid</u> — *"Do you feel hot when others don't?"*

Name / Age

PC - Empathy

SOCRATES——-------------------Impact

Is the patient stable?

Dizzy/ Faint

DDx S L i i M T

GIT Hx - Pan v BHT GaSY

P A M H U G S F O S S

S A D

Chronic Diarrhea

SOCRATES + **COCA-b** → if yes? Ask **BBL**

"Just to make sure there's nothing serious going on."

Celiac Ds / Colon CA/ Lymphoma / Stressors / Lactose Int / Infections / IBD / Meds / Thyroid

C C S L i i M T

DDx: *"I'd like to ask you a few questions to rule out other causes."*

Celiac Disease — *"Any allergy to bread?"*

Colon CA/ Lymphoma —*"Any hx of cancer? Any weight loss? Any lumps or bumps on their body?"*

Stressors — *"Any recent stressors or emotional news you got recently?"*

Lactose Intolerance —*"Are you lactose intolerant? Do you feel bloated or pass a lot of gas after consuming milk or dairy products?"*

Infection — *"Do you have a fever? Any hx of sick contacts? Any hx of travel? Any intake of street foods?"*

Inflammatory Bowel Disease (IBD) — *"Is there any blood in the stools?"* If yes, ask **BBL**. *"Any hx of joint pain? Hx of red eyes?"*

Medications – Abx/ Allergies — *"Are you on any medication? Which ones?"*

Name / Age

PC - Empathy

SOCRATES--------------------**Impact**

Is the patient dehydrated?

Dizzy/ faint

Weight loss

DDx C C S L i i M T

GIT Hx - Pan v BHT GaSY

P A M H U G S F O S S

|

S A D

Chronic Diarrhea (Continued)

Celiac Ds, Colon CA/ Lymphoma, Stressors, Lactose Int, Infections, IBD, Meds, Thyroid

C C S L i i M T

Thyroid — *"Do you feel hot or cold when others don't?"*

Name / Age

PC - Empathy

SOCRATES—-------------------**Impact**

Is the patient dehydrated?

Dizzy/ faint

Weight loss

SIGN POST DDx C C S L i i M T

GIT Hx - Pan v BHT GaSY

P A M H U G S F O S S

|

S A D

Bloody Diarrhea

SOCRATES + **COCA-b** → Ask **BBL**

SIGN POST *"Just to make sure there's nothing serious going on."*

Colitis, Hemorrhoids, Anal Fissures, Neoplasm, Diverticulitis, IBD

C H A N D I

SIGN POST DDx: *"I'd like to ask you a few questions to rule out other causes."*

<u>Colitis</u>:

- Infectious Colitis — *"Any associated fever? Any travel hx/ any sick contacts/ have you had any street food? Any hx of IV drug use? Needle sharing? Any hx of STIs? Hospitalization? Antibiotic abuse?"*
- Ischemic Colitis — *"Any abdominal pain after eating? Do you find that you are afraid to eat?"*

<u>Hemorrhoids</u> — *"Is the blood bright red? Is it present on the stool surface or toilet paper? Do you notice any lumps or swelling around the anus?"*

Name / Age

PC - Empathy

SOCRATES-------------------**Impact**

Is the patient stable?

Dizzy/faint

SIGN POST DDx C H A N D I

GIT Hx - Pan v BHT GaSY

P A M H U G S F O S S

S A D

Bloody Diarrhea (Continued)

Colitis / Hemorrhoids / Anal Fissures / Neoplasm / Diverticulitis / IBD

C H A N D I

Anal Fissures — *"Do you experience sharp pain during bowel movts? Did you notice any itching/* irritation around your 'anus/ bright red blood as a streak on stool surface rather than mixed in with stool?"

Neoplasm — *"Any hx of cancer? Any weight loss? Any lumps or bumps on your body?"*

Diverticulitis — *"Do you have associated LLQ abdominal pain?"*

Inflammatory Bowel Disease (IBD) — *"Is there any blood in the stools? Any hx of joint pain? Hx of red eyes?"*

Name / Age

PC - Empathy

SOCRATES—------------------**Impact**

Is the patient stable?

Dizzy/faint

SIGN POST DDx C H A N D I

GIT Hx - Pan v BHT GaSY

P A M   H U G S   F O S S

S A D

Acute Abdominal Pain

SOCRATES + Don't forget to ask SITE OF PAIN

SIGN POST *"Just to make sure there's nothing serious going on."*

Appendicitis, Intestinal Obs, Renal Colic, Pyelonephritis, Pancreatitis, Perforation, Aortic Dissection

A I R P P P AD

TOE P D M i A

SIGN POST DDx: *"I'd like to ask you a few questions to rule out other causes."*

Appendicitis – Site of pain → Central at first around the umbilicus then moves to the RLQ, associated with fever.

Intestinal Obstruction – Abdominal pain associated with nausea, vomiting, and bloody stools. *"Are you able to pass gas?"*

Renal Colic – Sharp abdominal pain can radiate to the groin, associated with bloody urine. Hx of kidney stones.

Pyelonephritis – Pain associated with fever/ burning micturition.

Pancreatitis — Pain worse on lying down and better on leaning forward. It may radiate to the back. May be associated with greasy stools.

Intestinal Perforation – Pt may have hx of peptic ulcer disease, heartburn, and a sour taste in the mouth. May have hx of recent NSAIDs or forceful vomiting.

Name / Age

PC - Empathy

SOCRATES———————————**Impact**

Trauma

Is the patient stable?

Dizzy/faint

SIGN POST DDx AIRPPPAD

TOE P

DMiA

GIT Hx - Pan v BHT GaSY

P A M H U G S F O S S

|

S A D

Acute Abdominal Pain (Continued)

Appendicitis, Intestinal Obs, Renal Colic, Pyelonephritis, Pancreatitis, Perforation, Aortic Dissection

A I R P P P AD

TOE P DMiA

Aortic Dissection — Sharp tearing pain radiating to the back.

Testicular torsion, Orchitis, Epididymitis, Prostatitis

Male: T O E P

Pain radiation to the groin. Ask about fever, redness, and swelling. Any hx of STIS/sexual history/ difficulty or burning in micturition.

Torsion (Ovarian), Ovarian Rupture, Ectopic Pregnancy, PID

Female: T O E P

Pain radiation to the groin. Ask about fever, redness, and swelling. LMP. Any hx of STIS/ sexual history/ burning in micturition.

For DMiA Check Elderly Abdominal Pain

Name / Age

PC - Empathy

SOCRATES——————————**Impact**

Trauma

Is the patient stable?

Dizzy/faint

DDx AIRPPPAD

TOE P

DMiA

GIT Hx - Pan v BHT GaSY

P A M H U G S F O S S

S A D

Abdominal Pain — Elderly

SOCRATES + Don't forget to ask SITE OF PAIN

SIGN POST *"Just to make sure there's nothing serious going on."*

Diverticulitis, MI, Mesenteric Ischemia, Aortic Aneurysm, Appendicitis, Intestinal Obs, Renal Colic, Pyelonephritis, Pancreatitis, Perforation, Aortic Dissection

D M i A A I R P P P AD

SIGN POST DDx: *"I'd like to ask you a few questions to rule out other causes."*

<u>Diverticulitis</u> —Site of pain → LLQ. Associated with fever.

<u>Myocardial infarction</u> — Pt complains of Substernal pain, ↑ on exertion, possibly radiating to the left arm, SOB, relieved by NTG/aspirin (angina).

<u>Mesenteric Ischemia</u> — *"Is it associated with meals?"*

<u>Aortic Aneurysm</u> — *" Have you noticed a pulsating lump or mass in your abdomen? Pain feels like it's tearing or radiating from the back."*

Check Abdominal Pain for AIRPPPAD & TOEP

Name / Age

PC - Empathy

SOCRATES------------------------**Impact**

Trauma

Is the patient stable?

Dizzy/faint

SIGN POST DDx **AIRPPPAD**

TOE P

DMiA

GIT Hx - Pan v BHT GaSY

P A M   H U G S   F O S S

S A D

Chronic Abdominal Pain

SIGN POST "*Just to make sure there's nothing serious going on.*"

chronic Pancreatitis, Colon cancer, Celiac disease, Lactose intolerance, IBS, IBD, Intestinal ischemia, Drug induced, Diet induced, Chronic Hepatitis

P C C L i i i d d Hep

SIGN POST DDx: "*I'd like to ask you a few questions to rule out other causes.*"

Chronic Pancreatitis — "*Have you noticed your pain worsening after eating, especially fatty meals? Have you had greasy, foul-smelling stools?*"

Colon Cancer — "*Any hx of cancer? Any weight loss? Any lumps or bumps on their body?*"

Celiac disease — "*Any allergy to bread?*"

Lactose intolerance — "*Are you lactose intolerant? Do you feel bloated or pass a lot of gas after consuming milk or dairy products?*"

Irritable Bowel Syndrome (IBS) — Diagnosis of exclusion. "*Does the pain improve after bowel movements? Have you noticed periods of constipation and diarrhea in the past?*"

Inflammatory bowel disease (IBD) — "*Is there any blood in the stools?*" If yes, ask **BBL**. "*Any hx of joint pain? Hx of red eyes?*"

Name / Age

PC - Empathy

SOCRATES—------------------Impact

Hx of weight loss/ night sweats/ fever

Hx of cancer

F/hx of cancer

SIGN POST DDx **PCC Liiidd Hep**

GIT Hx - Pan v BHT GaSY

P A M H U G S F O S S

S A D

Chronic Abdominal Pain (Continued)

chronic Pancreatitis
Colon cancer
Celiac disease
Lactose intolerance
IBS
IBD
Intestinal ischemia
Drug induced
Diet induced
Chronic Hepatitis

P C C L i i i d d Hep

Intestinal ischemia — *"Do you experience abdominal pain after eating? Do you find that you are afraid to eat?"*

Drug-induced — Abx/ Allergies — *"Are you on any medication? Which ones?"*

Diet-induced — *"What is your diet like?"*

Chronic Hepatitis — *"Have you noticed yellowing of skin or eyes, dark urine, or pale stools? Have you any hx of blood transfusions, IV drug use or unprotected sex?"*

Name / Age

PC - Empathy

SOCRATES---------------------Impact

Hx of weight loss/ night sweats/ fever

Hx of cancer

F/hx of cancer

SIGN POST DDx PCC Liiidd Hep

GIT Hx - Pan v BHT GaSY

P A M H U G S F O S S

S A D

Bright Red Blood Per rectum (BRBPR)

SOCRATES + **COCA-b → BBL**

"Just to make sure there's nothing serious going on."

Colitis, Hemorrhoids, Anal Fissures, Neoplasm, Diverticulitis, IBD

C H A N D I

DDx: *"I'd like to ask you a few questions to rule out other causes."*

<u>Colitis</u>:

- Infectious Colitis — *"Any associated fever? Any travel hx/ any sick contacts? Have you had any street food? Any hx of IV drug use/ Needle sharing? Any hx of STIs? Hospitalization? Antibiotic abuse?"*
- Ischemic Colitis — *"Any abdominal pain after eating? Do you find that you are afraid to eat?"*

<u>Hemorrhoids</u> — *"Is the blood bright red? Is it present on the stool surface or toilet paper? Do you notice any lumps or swelling around the anus?"*

Name / Age

PC - Empathy

SOCRATES—-------------------Impact

Is the patient stable?

Dizzy/faint

Weight loss/night sweats/ fever

DDx **C H A N D I**

GIT Hx - Pan v BHT GaSY

P A M H U G S F O S S

S A D

Bright Red Blood Per rectum (BRBPR) (Continued)

Colitis, Hemorrhoids, Anal Fissures, Neoplasm, Diverticulitis, IBD

C H A N D I

Anal Fissures — *"Do you experience sharp pain during bowel movts? Did you notice any itching/ irritation around your anal region? Did you notice bright red blood as a streak on stool surface rather than mixed in with stool?"*

Neoplasm — *"Any hx of cancer? Any weight loss? Any lumps or bumps on your body?"*

Diverticulitis — *"Do you have associated LLQ abdominal pain?"*

Inflammatory Bowel Disease (IBD) — *"Is there any blood in the stools? Any hx of joint pain? Hx of red eyes?"*

Name / Age

PC - Empathy

SOCRATES———————————Impact

Is the patient stable?

Dizzy/faint

Weight loss/night sweats/ fever

SIGN POST DDx **C H A N D I**

GIT Hx - Pan v BHT GaSY

P A M   H U G S   F O S S

S A D

Dysphagia

SOCRATES + *"Where does it get stuck? Above the clavicle or below? Is there difficulty in swallowing liquids or both solids and liquids?"*

"Just to make sure there's nothing serious going on."

Zenker's diverticulum, Abscess, Neuro- MS /MG, Strictures, Esophagitis, Achalasia, Lymphoma, Esophageal CA, DES, FB

Z A N   S E A L E D   F

DDx: *"I'd like to ask you a few questions to rule out other causes."*

Zenker's diverticulum — *"Do you experience any regurgitation of undigested food after eating? Do you have a sensation that food is stuck in your throat? Any history of bad breath?"*

Peritonsillar abscess / Retropharyngeal abscess — *"Any fever? Do you experience severe throat pain? Difficulty opening your mouth? Have you noticed that your voice is more muffled or a 'hot potato' voice?"*

Multiple Sclerosis — Chronic relapsing (previous episodes), NWT, b/b vision/gait/speech issues, loss of balance, falls, and depression.

Myasthenia Gravis — *"Do you notice any tiredness at the end of the day? Any drooping of eyelids end of day?"*

Name / Age

PC - Empathy

SOCRATES——------------------Impact

Hoarseness

Drooling

SOB

DDx **ZAN SEALED F**

GIT Hx - Pan v BHT GaSY

P A M   H U G S   F O S S

S A D

Dysphagia (Continued)

Zenker's diverticulum, Abscess, Neuro- MS /MG, Strictures, Esophagitis, Achalasia, Lymphoma, Esophageal CA, DES, FB

ZAN SEALED F

Name / Age

PC - Empathy

SOCRATES--------------------Impact

Hoarseness

Drooling

SOB

SIGN POST DDx ZAN SEALED F

GIT Hx - Pan v BHT GaSY

P A M   H U G S   F O S S

S A D

Parkinson's disease — *"Do you have a tremor when you are resting? Is it like a pin-rolling tremor? Do you find you have stiffness or rigidity when you move your arms or legs?"* – Shuffling gait. Difficult to initiate movement.

Stroke — *"Did you notice any issues with balance/with your eyes? Any blurring of vision? Any drooping of the face? Any weakness in the arm/leg?"*

Achalasia — *"Did you have difficulty with both solids and liquids from the start? Do you ever regurgitate undigested food when you lie down or at night?"*

Scleroderma — *"Have you noticed your fingers are thickened or stiff? Have they ever turned blue when exposed to cold?"*

Strictures — *"Any history of heartburn or acid reflux? Any hx of radiation to the throat? Do you have difficulty swallowing solids only or at first?"*

Esophagitis — *"Do you experience pain or a burning sensation when swallowing? Are you on any immunosuppressants?"*

Dysphagia (Continued)

Zenker's diverticulum, Abscess, Neuro- MS /MG, Strictures, Esophagitis, Achalasia, Lymphoma, Esophageal CA, DES, FB

ZAN SEALED F

Lymphoma /Esophageal CA — *"Was there a progressive deterioration, with the first difficulty in swallowing solids and then both solids and liquids?"*

Diffuse esophageal Spasm — *"Do you experience intermittent chest pain along with your swallowing difficulty? Have you noticed this being triggered by stress or hot/cold food or liquids?"*

Foreign Body — *"Did this happen suddenly after eating or swallowing something, like a piece of meat or a small object?"*

Name / Age

PC - Empathy

SOCRATES—-------------------Impact

Hoarseness

Drooling

SOB

SIGN POST DDx ZAN SEALED F

GIT Hx - Pan v BHT GaSY

P A M H U G S F O S S

S A D

Jaundice

SIGN POST "*Just to make sure there's nothing serious going on.*"

PBC/Pregnant, Hemolysis, Hepatitis, Fatty liver, TB, Sepsis, Meds, Alcohol, Cirrhosis, Cholangitis, Cholecystitis, Pancreatitis, Cholangio CA, Pancreatic CA

PHHFTS! MAC C P-CA

SIGN POST DDx: "*I'd like to ask you a few questions to rule out other causes.*"

Pregnant / Primary Biliary cirrhosis (PBC) — "*Are you by any chance pregnant? When was your last LMP? Have you noticed any associated itching on your palms and soles? Any h/x of thyroid disease or autoimmune diseases?*"

Hemolysis — "*Do you have a h/x of anemia, fatigue or recent infections? Have you noticed your urine is darker in colour, especially in the morning?*"

Hepatitis — "*Any associated fever? Have you any hx of blood transfusions, IV drug use or unprotected sex?*"

Fatty Liver — "*Do you have a h/x of obesity/ diabetes/ High cholesterol/ High blood pressure? Have you noticed fatigue and weight changes?*"

TB/Sepsis — "*Do you have a fever? Any hx of sick contacts? Any hx of travel?*"

Name / Age

PC - Empathy

SOCRATES—------------------Impact

Disoriented/ Confused pt

SIGN POST DDx **P H H F T S!**

MAC CP-CA

GIT Hx - Pan v BHT GaSY

P A M   H U G S   F O S S

S A D

Jaundice (Continued)

PBC/Pregnant, Hemolysis, Hepatitis, Fatty liver, TB, Sepsis, Meds, Alcohol, Cirrhosis, Cholangitis, Cholecystitis, Pancreatitis, Cholangio CA, Pancreatic CA

PHHFTS! MAC C P-CA

Medications — *"Are you on any medications? What is the Dosage/duration?"* — Remember ***"I AM CHAT PRiFS"*** (Isoniazid, Acetaminophen, Methotrexate, Chlorpromazine, Herbal Chinese bush tea, Amiodarone, Tetracyclines, Phenytoin, Rifampicin, Antifungal (ketoconazole), Statins & Sulfa drugs)

Alcohol — *"Do you drink alcohol? How many glasses per day? For how long?"*

Cirrhosis — *"Any hx of chronic liver disease? Have you noticed any swelling in your legs? In your abdomen (ascites)? Any hx of easy bruising or bleeding?"*

Cholangitis/Cholecystitis — *"Any fever/ nausea or vomiting? Any RUQ pain after eating fatty foods?"*

Pancreatitis — Pain worse on lying down and better on leaning forward. It may radiate to the back. May be associated with greasy stools.

Cholangiocarcinoma/ Pancreatic carcinoma — Painless jaundice. *"Any hx of cancer? Any weight loss? Any lumps or bumps on their body?"*

Name / Age

PC - Empathy

SOCRATES-------------------Impact

Disoriented/ Confused pt

SIGN POST

DDx P H H F T S!
MAC CP-CA

GIT Hx - Pan v BHT GaSY

P A M   H U G S   F O S S

S A D

Urinary System

How to organise yourself before entering the station + KEY **178**

Hematuria **182**

Urinary incontinence **184**

Stress Incontinence. **186**

Erectile Dysfunction. **217**

Penile Discharge .... Error! Bookmark not defined.

Benign Prostatic Hyperplasia (BPH) **190**

Lower UTI. .... Error! Bookmark not defined.

Renal Colic. **193**

Lymphadenopathy. **195**

Scrotal Mass. **197**

How to organise yourself before entering the station

Before entering the station, you will have under two minutes to read the prompt and jot down notes in your booklet.

These notes should focus on key information you'll need to remember while taking the history from the standardized participant (SP). The SP is an actor trained to portray a specific medical condition or scenario. Their purpose is to interact with you and allow the physician examiner (PE) to observe and assess your performance.

The booklet provided is rectangular, about half the size of an A4 sheet. It contains blank sheets for your notes, as well as candidate code stickers, which you'll need to hand over to the examiner before starting each station.

Given the time constraints and anxiety during the station, these notes can serve as a valuable guide to help you complete a thorough history.

Therefore, it is essential to practice responding to prompts and mastering the '2-minute drill' regularly to achieve your best results.

HOW TO PRACTICE :

For practice purposes, folding an A4 sheet in half works well to simulate the booklet.

Hence, this book is divided into two columns:

Left column	**Right column**
Contains a breakdown of the mnemonics and the questions you may need to ask.	Notes to write in your booklet as part of your 2-minute drill, often including mnemonics that make the best use of your time and help you recall essential steps efficiently!

These structured notes will provide a clear and concise roadmap to ensure you stay focused and efficient during the station.

The KEY

Knock on the door, Walk in, Wear a smile, Greet the examiner, and hand the candidate code, "*Hi, here's my candidate code.*"
Sanitize your hands and simultaneously:

Introduce yourself to the standardized participant (SP):
"Hello, I am Dr____ and I will be your physician today. May I know your name and age, please? How would you like to be addressed? That's great!

"Is it okay if I sit down and take a few notes?"

PC: Presenting Complaints
"What brings you in here today?"
Listen to the patient. It is important to express **Empathy.**
"I am sorry to hear that. That must be quite distressing."

"Okay, so I would like to ask you a few questions and do a physical exam after, and we will figure out a treatment plan for you today!"

SOCRATES-B: For conditions with other symptoms, SOCRATES-B can still be used.

- site: *"Where is the pain? Can you point at it?"*
- onset: *"Was it gradual or sudden in onset?"*
- character: *"What kind of pain is it? Is it a dull pain or a sharp pain?"*
- radiate: *"Does the pain radiate anywhere?"*
- associated symptoms: *"Any associated symptoms?"*
- time: *"Is the pain constant or intermittent?"*
- exacerbating factor: *"Does anything relieve the pain or make it worse?"*
- severity: *"On a scale from 1-10, how would you rate the pain? 10 being the worst."*
- before: *"Have you had this before?"*

Not every P/C involves pain. Some complaints may just require 'o-ate' onset associated s/s, time, and exacerbating/ relieving factors.

COCA-b: For any vomiting/discharge/sputum/stool/urine.
Colour, **O**dor, **C**onsistency, **A**mount, **B**lood (If yes for blood, ask **BBL**)

BBL — (if pt complains of bleeding), stands for :

- Blood thinners – *"Are you on blood thinners?"*
- Bloody Diarrhea – *"Do you bruise easily or bleed easily?"*
- Liver Disease — *"Any hx of liver disease?"*

Impact: *"How are you coping with this?"*

DDX: Differentials for the condition given for each condition.

SIGNPOST: This symbol means you have to signpost! A signpost is an introductory statement. This is to introduce your segment of questions so the examiner is aware of your line of questioning.

E.g.: DDx - means you have to place an introductory statement before asking for differentials: *"I am going to ask a few questions to rule out any other causes."*

Red flags: This is for conditions we need to rule out right away as they may require urgent attention.

PAM HUGS FOSS: stands for:

- Past medical hx: *"Since this is the first time we are meeting, do you have any past medical conditions that I should know about? Or that you have been treated for?"*
- Allergies: *"Do you have any allergies?"*
- Medications: *"Are you on any medications? What are the medications? Are you adherent with your medications? What is the dosage?"*
- Hospitalization/Surgery: *"Have you ever been hospitalized before? Any surgeries done before?"*
- Urinary changes: *"Have you noticed changes in your urine?"*
- GIT changes: *"Have you noticed any changes in your bowel habits?"*
- SAD- **S**moking/**A**lcohol/Recreational **D**rugs:
    - *"Do you smoke? How many cigarettes a day? For how long? Have you ever thought about quitting?"*
    - *"Do you drink alcohol? How often?"*
    - *"Have you done any recreational drugs? What have you used? How do you take it? Do you sniff or inject? Do you share needles?"*
- Family history: *"Any family history of any medical conditions?"* Specific medical conditions you are concerned about.
- Occupation: *"If I may ask, what do you do for a living?"*
- Social: *"May I know about your living conditions? Who do you live with?"*
- Support: *"Do you have any family around? Are they supportive? That's good to know."*

Mnemonics for system questions:
Urology hx:

B²P FUNDS

- Bleeding
- Burning
- Pain on pee/ejaculation
- Frequency
- Urgency
- Nocturia
- Discharge
- Stones

SHED MC for voiding symptoms

- Straining
- Hesitancy
- a feeling of incomplete Emptying
- Dribbling
- Medications
- Hx of Catheterization

Hematuria

SOCRATES + **COCA-b** → ask **BBL**

SIGN POST "*Just to make sure there's nothing serious going on.*"

Infection, Interstitial GN, Tumor, Stone, HUS, Exercise, Meds, Occupation, Trauma, Sickle cell ds/SLE, Diet

i i t 's h e m o t s d

SIGN POST DDx: "*I'd like to ask you a few questions to rule out other causes.*"

Infection — "*Do you have a fever? Any hx of sick contacts? Any hx of travel? Any intake of street foods recently?*"

Interstitial Glomerulonephritis — "*Have you had any recent fever? Swelling in your face or body?*" (drug-induced GN is a common cause so you can also ask about drug history).

Tumor —"*Any hx of cancer? Any weight loss? Any lumps or bumps on their body?*"

Kidney stones —"*Any associated pain with the bloody urine? Any hx of kidney disease or kidney stones?*"

Hemolytic Uremic Syndrome (HUS) — "*Have you had any recent episodes of bloody diarrhea? Have you noticed that you are paler or weaker recently? Have they had any unexplained bruising?*"

Name / Age

PC - Empathy

SOCRATES—-----------------Impact

Trauma

Abdominal/ groin Pain

Weight loss, night sweats, fever

Ask **BBL**:

- Blood thinners – "*Are you on blood thinners?*"
- Blood disorders – "*Do you bruise easily or bleed easily?*"
- Liver Disease — "*Any hx of liver disease?*"

SIGN POST DDx iit's hemots d

Uro Hx -B^{2}P FUNDS

P A M H U G S F O S S

|

S A D

Hematuria (Continued)

Infection, Interstitial GN, Tumor, Stone, HUS, Exercise, Meds, Occupation, Trauma, Sickle cell ds/SLE, Diet

i i t ' s h e m o t s d

Exercise — *"Have you recently engaged in intense physical activity? Did you notice the blood in your urine right after exercising? And does it clear with rest and hydration?"*

Medications — *"Are you on any medications? What is the Dosage/duration?"*

Occupation — *"What do you do for a living? Have you ever worked in an industrial area like a rubber, steel, or chemical factory?"*

Trauma — *"Did you hurt yourself?"*

Systemic Lupus Erythematosus (SLE) — *"Have you noticed any rashes on your face or body? Have you experienced sensitivity to light? Have you noticed that your skin is paler than others? Have you had any oral ulcers? Any weakness/ fatigue/ fever?"*

Diet — *"What is your diet like? Have you eaten any food like beetroots or berries recently"*

Name / Age

PC - Empathy

SOCRATES———————————Impact

Trauma

Abdominal/ groin Pain

Weight loss, night sweats, fever

Ask **BBL**:

- Blood thinners – *"Are you on blood thinners?"*
- Blood disorders – *"Do you bruise easily or bleed easily?"*
- Liver Disease — *"Any hx of liver disease?"*

SIGN POST DDx **iit's hemots d**

Uro Hx -B^{2}P FUNDS

P A M H U G S F O S S

|

S A D

Urinary incontinence

"*Just to make sure there's nothing serious going on.*"

Spinal Cord Lesion, **NPH**, Infection, Parkinson's ds, Stroke, DM, Alzheimer's ds, Constipation, Caffeine, Meds, MS

S h i p s d a c c m m

DDx: "*I'd like to ask you a few questions to rule out other causes.*"

Spinal cord lesion — "*Any N.W.T in your legs? Have issues with your bowel movements? Do you feel it when you wipe?*"

Normal Pressure Hydrocephalus (NPH) — "*Do you have difficulty walking? Have you experienced any changes in memory/ any confusion/ or difficulty concentrating?*"

Infection —"*Do you have a fever? Any hx of sick contacts? Any hx of travel? Any intake of street foods recently?*"

Parkinson's disease — "*Do you have a tremor when you are resting? Is it like a pin-rolling tremor? Do you find you have stiffness or rigidity when you move your arms or legs?*"

Stroke — **BE FAST**

Diabetes Mellitus (DM) — "*Have you noticed you have been peeing a lot/been thirsty a lot? Have you been diagnosed with diabetes? Any f/hx of diabetes?*"

Name / Age

PC - Empathy

SOCRATES—------------------Impact

Trauma

Constitution s/s

b/b

N.W.T

BE FAST

DDx **Ships dacc mm**

Uro Hx -B²P FUNDS

P A M   H U G S   F O S S

|

S A D

Urinary Incontinence (Continued)

Spinal Cord Lesion, NPH, Infection, Parkinson's ds, Stroke, DM, Alzheimer's ds, Constipation, Caffeine, Meds, MS

S h i p s d a c c m m

<u>Alzheimer's disease</u> — *"Have you noticed any decline in your memory? Are you forgetting words/ numbers/ names/ recent events or remote events?"*

<u>Constipation</u> — *"Do you have constipation?"*

<u>Caffeine</u> — *"Do you drink a lot of coffee?"*

<u>Medications</u> — *"Are you taking any medications?"* If yes, ask about dosage/duration.

<u>Multiple Sclerosis</u> — Chronic relapsing (previous episodes), NWT, b/b vision/gait/speech issues, loss of balance, falls, also depression.

Name / Age

PC - Empathy

SOCRATES——------------------Impact

Trauma

Constitution s/s

b/b

N.W.T

BE FAST

DDx **Ships dacc mm**

Uro Hx -B^{2}P FUNDS

P A M H U G S F O S S

|

S A D

Stress Incontinence

SIGN POST "*Just to make sure there's nothing serious going on.*"

Causes: C p h o d (Chronic Cough, Pregnancy, Hysterectomy, Obesity, Multiple Deliveries)

Chronic cough — "*Do you have a chronic cough? Or any conditions like asthma or lung disease? Do you smoke? Any history or sour taste in your mouth? Do you take any medications?" (ACE inhibitors)*

Pregnancy /Multiple deliveries — "*Have you had any pregnancies or vaginal deliveries?*"

Hysterectomy – "*Have you had any surgeries like hysterectomy or pelvic floor procedures?*"

Obesity— "*Have you noticed any recent weight gain? Have you been told that you have obesity?*"

S h i p s d a c c m m (Spinal Cord Lesion, **NPH**, Infection, Parkinson's ds, Stroke, DM, Alzheimer's ds, Constipation, Caffeine, Meds, MS)

SIGN POST DDx: "*I'd like to ask you a few questions to rule out other causes.*"

(Check Urinary Incontinence)

Name / Age

PC - Empathy

SOCRATES——————————**Impact**

Is the patient dehydrated

Dizzy/faint

Causes: C p h o d

SIGN POST DDx Ships dacc mm

Uro Hx -B^{2}P FUNDS

P A M H U G S F O S S

|

S A D

Erectile Dysfunction

Substances, Psychogenic, Insufficiency of Blood, Neurological, Endocrine, Abnormal Curved Penis, Trauma

S P I N E A T

DDx: *"I'd like to ask you a few questions to rule out other causes."*

Substances — *"Have you recently started any new medications for blood pressure, depression, or other conditions?"*

Psychogenic — *"Have you been feeling stressed or anxious? If I may ask, are you having relationship difficulties? Do you still experience morning erections?"*

Insufficiency of Blood — *"Do you have a history of high blood pressure? Or high cholesterol? Or heart disease? Do you have leg pain while walking that improves with rest?"*

Neurological — *"Have you had any N.W.T in your legs or hands? Do you have diabetes? If yes, how well is your blood sugar controlled?"*

Endocrine — *"Have you noticed a decrease in muscle mass? Energy? Sex drive? Have you noticed any nipple discharge? Do you feel cold when others don't?"*

Name / Age

PC - Empathy

SOCRATES--------------------**Impact**

DDx **SPINE AT**

Uro Hx -B^2P FUNDS

P A M H U G S F O S S

S A D

Erectile Dysfunction (Continued)

Substances — Psychogenic — Insufficiency of Blood — Neurological — Endocrine — Abnormal Curved Penis — Trauma

S P I N E A T

Abnormal Curved Penis — *"If I may ask, have you noticed a curve or bend in your penis, especially when erect?"*

Trauma — *"Have you had any injuries to your pelvic area, such as a fall? Or had prostate surgery? Any radiation treatment?"*

Name / Age

PC - Empathy

SOCRATES——————————**Impact**

DDx **S P I N E A T**

Uro Hx -B^{2}P FUNDS

P A M H U G S F O S S

S A D

Penile Discharge

SOCRATES + **COCA-b**

"Is it associated with: itching, fever, lesions on genitalia, ulcers on genitalia or mouth, rash, abdominal pain, or hx of UTIs?"

Ask "**I flura u**"

Ask about Risky Behavior:

MSM
Age of Intercourse
Multiple Sexual partners
Unprotected Sex
Hx of STIs
IVDU

M A S S Hx I

Remember →May need to <u>Report</u>

→Treat sexual partners

Name / Age

PC - Empathy

SOCRATES—-------------------Impact

Associated s/s - **I Flura U**

COCA-B

CONFIDENTIALITY

Uro Hx -B^2P FUNDS

+ Risky Behaviour - **"MASSHi"**

If adolescents ask **HEADSS**

P A M H U G S F O S S

|

S A D

Benign Prostatic Hyperplasia (BPH)

"Just to make sure there's nothing serious going on."

Uro Hx -B^{2}P FUNDS + **SHED MC**

Spinal Cord Lesion, **NPH**, Infection, Parkinson's ds, Stroke, DM, Alzheimer's ds, Constipation, Caffeine, Meds, MS

S h i p s d a c c m m

DDx: *"I'd like to ask you a few questions to rule out other causes."*

(Check Urinary Incontinence)

Name / Age

PC - Empathy

SOCRATES——-------------------Impact

Constitution s/s

B/b

N.w.t

Difficulty walking

Uro Hx - B^{2}P FUNDS + SHED MC

DDx Ships dacc mm

P A M   H U G S   F O S S

S A D

Lower UTI

SOCRATES + **COCA-b**

Stone Infection Trauma Tumor Meds BPH

S i t t m b

SIGN POST DDx: *"I'd like to ask you a few questions to rule out other causes."*

Stone — *"Any hx of kidney disease? "Do you have severe flank pain that comes and goes? or radiates to the groin? Have you noticed blood in your urine?"*

Infection — *"Do you have burning pain while urinating or urgency to go? Have you had a fever? chills? or lower abdominal pain?"*

Trauma — *"Have you had any recent falls, pelvic injuries, or surgeries? Did your symptoms start after an accident or direct impact to your lower abdomen?"*

Name / Age

PC - Empathy

SOCRATES——-------------------Impact

SIGN POST DDx Sittmb

Uro Hx -B^{2}P FUNDS

P A M H U G S F O S S

|

S A D

Lower UTI (Continued)

Stone Infection Trauma Tumor Meds BPH

S i t t m b

Tumor — *"Have you noticed blood in your urine without any pain? Have you had any unexplained weight loss or night sweats?"*

Medication — *"Have you recently started any new medications for blood pressure or overactive bladder? Do you take diuretics or any medications that increase urination?"*

Benign Prostatic Hyperplasia (BPH) — *"Do you have a weak urine stream? Difficulty starting urination, or feel like your bladder isn't emptying completely? Do you wake up multiple times at night to urinate?"*

Name / Age

PC - Empathy

SOCRATES—-------------------Impact

SIGN POST DDx **S i t t m b**

Uro Hx -B^2P FUNDS

P A M H U G S F O S S

S A D

Renal Colic

SIGN POST *"Just to make sure there's nothing serious going on."*

Kidney Diet Meds UTI Dehydration Parathyroid

Ki d m u d PTH

SIGN POST DDx: *"I'd like to ask you a few questions to rule out other causes."*

Kidney — *"Any hx of kidney disease? Have you noticed blood in your urine?"*

Diet — *"Do you consume a lot of high-salt or high-protein foods, like processed foods or red meat? Do you drink a lot of tea, spinach, or nuts?"* (which are high in oxalates)

Medication — *"Are you taking any supplements like calcium or vitamin C? Have you recently started any new medications, such as diuretics or antibiotics?"*

Urinary Tract Infection (UTI) — *"Do you have burning pain while urinating or a frequent urge to go? Have you had a fever, chills, or nausea along with your pain?"*

Name / Age

PC - Empathy

SOCRATES—------------------Impact

Trauma

RF: **Kid mud PTH**

Uro Hx -B^{2}P FUNDS

P A M H U G S F O S S

|

S A D

Renal Colic (Continued)

Kidney Diet Meds UTI Dehydration Parathyroid

Ki d m u d PTH

<u>Dehydration</u> — *"How much water do you typically drink in a day? Have you had episodes of excessive sweating, vomiting, or diarrhea recently?"*

<u>PTH</u> — *"Have you had a history of recurrent kidney stones? Have you experienced bone pain, fatigue, muscle weakness, or frequent fractures?"*

Name / Age

PC - Empathy

SOCRATES———————————Impact

Trauma

RF: **Kid mud PTH**

Uro Hx -B^{2}P FUNDS

P A M H U G S F O S S

|

S A D

Lymphadenopathy

SIGN POST *"Just to make sure there's nothing serious going on."*

Leukemia/ Lymphoma, Sarcoidosis, Toxo, Infection, Travel hx, Cat scratch ds, HIV, Mononucleosis, Cancers

L s t i t c h Mo C

SIGN POST DDx: *"I'd like to ask you a few questions to rule out other causes."*

Leukemia/ Lymphoma — *"Have you noticed unexplained weight loss or night sweats? Persistent fatigue? Do you have painless nodes on your body?"*

Sarcoidosis — *"Have you had a chronic cough? Shortness of breath? or skin rashes? Have you ever been diagnosed with an autoimmune disease?"*

Toxoplasmosis — *"Have you recently eaten undercooked meat? Do you own a cat? Have you had flu-like symptoms such as fever? or muscle aches? or swollen glands?"*

Infection — *"Have you had any recent sore throat, fever, or skin infections?"*

Travel hx — *"Have you travelled recently?"* Ask about the location of travel to check if it was to regions that have high rates of tuberculosis or parasitic infections.

Name / Age

PC - Empathy

SOCRATES—-------------------Impact

Weight loss, night sweats, fever

SIGN POST DDx **L stitch MoC**

P A M H U G S F O S S

|

S A D

Lymphadenopathy (Continued)

Leukemia/ Lymphoma
Sarcoidosis
Toxo
Infection
Travel hx
Cat scratch ds
HIV
Mononucleosis
Cancers

L s t i t c h Mo C

Cat Scratch Disease — *"Have you been scratched or bitten by a cat recently? Do you have red, swollen skin near the scratch site?"*

HIV — Ask about sexual history. *"Have you had any recent unprotected sexual contact? Any blood transfusions? or needle sharing? Have you experienced unexplained fevers or mouth sores? or night sweats?"*

Mononucleosis — *"Have you had a sore throat? or swollen tonsils? Did your symptoms start after close contact with someone who was sick?"*

Cancers — *"Have you had difficulty swallowing? Hoarseness, or persistent cough? Have you noticed any lumps or bumps on your body?"*

Name / Age

PC - Empathy

SOCRATES—-------------------Impact

Weight loss, night sweats, fever

SIGN POST DDx L stitch MoC

P A M H U G S F O S S

S A D

Scrotal Mass

"Just to make sure there's nothing serious going on."

Testicular Torsion — Orchitis — Epididymitis

T O E

DDx: *"I'd like to ask you a few questions to rule out other causes."*

Testicular Torsion — Torsion pain is acute and intense. *"Does the pain get worse when you lift the scrotum?"* (Negative Prehn's sign: pain does not improve with elevation in torsion.)

Orchitis — *"Have you recently had a fever, mumps, or a viral illness? Is the pain gradually worsening with redness or swelling in the scrotum?"*

Epididymitis — *"Did the pain start gradually and does it improve when you lift the scrotum? Have you had any burning sensation when urinating?"* Get a sexual history to ask about any recent unprotected sexual contact.

Name / Age

PC - Empathy

SOCRATES——-------------------Impact

Painful Mass

Trauma

DDx

Painful: T O E

Painless: H E S T V

Uro Hx -B^2P FUNDS

P A M H U G S F O S S

S A D

Scrotal Mass (Continued)

Testicular Torsion   Orchitis   Epididymitis

T O E

<u>Hydrocele</u> — *"Does the swelling change in size throughout the day? or when lying down? Is the mass soft?"*

<u>Epididymal Cyst</u> — *"Have you noticed that it is separate from your testicle? Do you have any history of scrotal trauma or infections?"*

<u>Spermatocele</u> — *"Does the lump feel like a fluid-filled sac near the top of your testicle? Have you had a vasectomy or any scrotal surgeries?"*

<u>Testicular Tumor</u> — *"Have you noticed any changes in the size or shape of your testicle? Do you find that the mass is firm and hard? Have you experienced unexplained weight loss?"*

<u>Varicocele</u> — *"Does the swelling feel like a 'bag of worms' when you touch it? Does the swelling decrease when you lie down? Is it worse when standing or straining?"*

Name / Age

PC - Empathy

SOCRATES—-------------------Impact

Painful Mass

Trauma

SIGN POST DDx

Painful: **T O E**

Painless: **H E S T V**

Uro Hx -B^{2}P FUNDS

P A M   H U G S   F O S S

S A D

Neurology

How to organise yourself before entering the station + KEY 200

Headache. 204

Tremors 207

Parkinson's Disease 209

Dizziness/Vertigo 210

Gait 212

Concussions 214

Seizures 215

Stroke 217

Subarachnoid Hemorrhage 218

Sleep Apnea 219

Facial Palsy 221

Hoarseness 223

Multiple Sclerosis 225

How to organise yourself before entering the station

Before entering the station, you will have under two minutes to read the prompt and jot down notes in your booklet.

These notes should focus on key information you'll need to remember while taking the history from the standardized participant (SP). The SP is an actor trained to portray a specific medical condition or scenario. Their purpose is to interact with you and allow the physician examiner (PE) to observe and assess your performance.

The booklet provided is rectangular, about half the size of an A4 sheet. It contains blank sheets for your notes, as well as candidate code stickers, which you'll need to hand over to the examiner before starting each station.

Given the time constraints and anxiety during the station, these notes can serve as a valuable guide to help you complete a thorough history.

Therefore, it is essential to practice responding to prompts and mastering the '2-minute drill' regularly to achieve your best results.

HOW TO PRACTICE :

For practice purposes, folding an A4 sheet in half works well to simulate the booklet.

Hence this book is divided into two columns:

Left column	Right column
Contains a breakdown of the mnemonics and the questions you may need to ask.	Notes to write in your booklet as part of your 2-minute drill, often including mnemonics that make the best use of your time and help you recall essential steps efficiently!

These structured notes will provide a clear and concise roadmap to ensure you stay focused and efficient during the station.

The KEY

Knock on the door, Walk in, Wear a smile, Greet the examiner, and hand the candidate code, *"Hi, here's my candidate code."*
Sanitize your hands and simultaneously:

Introduce yourself to the standardized participant (SP):
"Hello, I am Dr___ and I will be your physician today. May I know your name and age, please? How would you like to be addressed? That's great!

"Is it okay if I sit down and take a few notes?"

PC: Presenting Complaints
"What brings you in here today?"
Listen to the patient. It is important to express **Empathy.**
"I am sorry to hear that. That must be quite distressing."

"Okay, so I would like to ask you a few questions and do a physical exam after and we will figure out a treatment plan for you today!"

SOCRATES-B: For conditions with other symptoms SOCRATES-B can still be used.

- site: *"Where is the pain? Can you point at it?"*
- onset: *"Was it gradual or sudden in onset?"*
- character: *"What kind of pain is it? Is it a dull pain or a sharp pain?"*
- radiate: *"Does the pain radiate anywhere?"*
- associated symptoms: *"Any associated symptoms?"*
- time: *"Is the pain constant or intermittent?"*
- exacerbating factor: *"Does anything relieve the pain or make it worse?"*
- severity: *"On a scale from 1-10, how would you rate the pain? 10 being the worst."*
- before: *"Have you had this before?"*

Not every P/C involves pain. Some complaints may just require 'o-ate' onset associated s/s, time, and exacerbating/ relieving factors.

COCA-b: For any vomiting/discharge/sputum/stool/urine.
Colour, **O**dor, **C**onsistency, **A**mount, **B**lood (If yes for blood , ask **BBL**)

BBL — (if pt complains of bleeding), stands for :

- Blood thinners – *"Are you on blood thinners?"*
- Bloody Diarrhea – *"Do you bruise easily or bleed easily?"*
- Liver Disease — *"Any hx of liver disease?"*

Impact: *"How are you coping with this?"*

DDX: Differentials for the condition given for each condition.

SIGNPOST: This symbol means you have to signpost! A signpost is an introductory statement. This is to introduce your segment of questions so the examiner is aware of your line of questioning.

E.g.: DDx - means you have to place an introductory statement before asking for differentials: *"I am going to ask a few questions to rule out any other causes."*

Red flags: This is for conditions we need to rule out right away as they may require urgent attention.

PAM HUGS FOSS: stands for:

- Past medical hx: *"Since this is the first time we are meeting, do you have any past medical conditions that I should know about? Or that you have been treated for?"*
- Allergies: *"Do you have any allergies?"*
- Medications: *"Are you on any medications? What are the medications? Are you adherent with your medications? What is the dosage?"*
- Hospitalization/Surgery: *"Have you ever had any hospitalization before? Any surgeries done before?"*
- Urinary changes: *"Have you noticed changes in your urine?"*
- GIT changes: *"Have you noticed any changes in your bowel habits?"*
- SAD - **S**moking/**A**lcohol/Recreational **D**rugs:
    - *"Do you smoke? How many cigarettes a day? For how long? Have you ever thought about quitting?"*
    - *"Do you drink alcohol? How often?"*
    - *"Have you done any recreational drugs? What have you used? How do you take it? Do you sniff or inject? Do you share needles?"*
- Family history: *"Any family history of any medical conditions?"* Specific medical conditions you are concerned about.
- Occupation: *"If I may ask, what do you do for a living?"*
- Social: *"May I know about your living conditions? Who do you live with?"*
- Support: *"Do you have any family around? Are they supportive? That's good to know."*

Mnemonics for system questions:
Neurological hx

HV LWN BCSSS - (SAM)

- Headache – "
- Visual disturbances
- LOC
- **NWT** – Numbness, Weakness, Tingling
- Balance
- Change in taste, smell, hearing
- Speech difficulty
- Swallowing difficulty
- Seizures
- Sleep Change
- Activities
- Mood Change

BE FAST:

- Balance/ Eye issues FAST –*"Did you notice any issues with balance/with your eyes? Any blurring of vision?"*
- Facial droop/ Arm weakness – *"Any drooping of face? Any weakness of arm/leg?"*
- Swallowing/speech issues – *"Any difficulty swallowing? Or speaking?"*
- Time to call 911/ go to ER (If all positive Time to call 911/ go to ER → Alert stroke code

Headache

SIGN POST *"Just to make sure there's nothing serious going on."*

neural Deficits, upon Awakening, Fever, Thunderclap headache, New Headache, Neck Stiffness, on Exertion, Scalp Tenderness, Seizures

D a f t n e s s

Primary Headache:

Migraine, Tension, Cluster

M T C

SIGN POST DDx: *"I'd like to ask you a few questions to rule out other causes."*

Migraine — Unilateral, throbbing headache. Associated symptoms include: aura, photophobia, and phonophobia.

Tension Headache — Band-like headache. Ask about stressors and poor posture.

Cluster Headache — Associated with ipsilateral nasal congestion, and ptosis.

Secondary Headache:

Temporal Arteritis, ↑ICP, Tumor, SAH, Meningitis/ Enceph, Others*

T i t s MO

Name / Age

PC - Empathy

SOCRATES——-------------------Impact

▶D a f t n e s s

SIGN POST DDx

Primary headache: M T C

Secondary headache: T i T S MO (hotdogs LMP) ↲

Neuro Hx — HV LWN BCSSS - SAM

P A M H U G S F O S S

S A D

Headache (Continued)

Secondary Headache:

Temporal Arteritis / ↑ICP / Tumor / SAH / Meningitis/ Enceph / Others*

T i t s MO

SIGN POST DDx: *"I'd like to ask you a few questions to rule out other causes."*

Temporal Arteritis — ↑50 years of age. Pt experiences pain when combing hair, chewing, and getting out of bed. *"Do you experience scalp tenderness? "When you touch your temples, is it painful? Do you feel a cord-like structure there? Any blurry vision? fever? chills? jaw pain?"*

↑ICP — (↑BP ↓HR tachypnea) Headache is constant! Worse in the a.m., worse when supine/ worse with the Valsalva maneuver. *"Do you have HTN? Have you recently checked your BP? Do you have blurry vision?"* Ask about salty food intake/ f/x./Hx of tumour, trauma/ fall.

Tumor — Ask about **NWT**, and neural deficits. Remember Prolactinoma – can occur in young pts.

Meningitis/ Enceph — *"Any fever? neck stiffness? chills? nausea/vomiting? confusion? LOC? Any rashes?"*

Name / Age

PC - Empathy

SOCRATES--------------------Impact

▶ D a f t n e s s

SIGN POST DDx

Primary headache: M T C

Secondary headache: T i T S MO (hotdogs LMP) ↲

Neuro Hx — HV LWN BCSSS - SAM

P A M H U G S F O S S

S A D

Headache (Continued)

Hypoxia, Optic Neuritis, Trauma, Dental Infection, OA of jaw/spine, Glaucoma, Sinusitis/ Mastoiditis, Lumbar Puncture, Meds overuse, Preeclampsia

H O T D O G S L M P

<u>Subarachnoid hemorrhage</u> (SAH) — Pt refers to this as the worst headache in life! Also referred to as a Thunderclap headache. Acute onset/ worst on exertion.

<u>Other</u> — **HOT DOGS LMP**

<u>There can be other causes of headaches-</u>

"Do you feel short of breath or have difficulty breathing? Have you been in high-altitude areas recently? Any hx of trauma? Or dental infection? Any pain with eye movement or vision issues? Any pain in the jaw? Do you have a history of glaucoma or eye pressure issues? Any hx of sinus issues? Any hx of LP? Any change in dosage for the medications you have been taking lately?"

Name / Age

PC - Empathy

SOCRATES--------------------Impact

D a f t n e s s

DDx

Primary headache: **M T C**

Secondary headache: **T i T S MO**
(hotdogs LMP)

Neuro Hx — HV LWN BCSSS - SAM

P A M H U G S F O S S

S A D

Tremors

"Just to make sure there's nothing serious going on."

b/b — *"Any bladder and bowel changes?"*

NWT — *"Any numbness, weakness or tingling of any part of your body?"*

BE FAST — Qs to rule out stroke (Refer to Key)

At Rest/ Intentional tremor:

Parkinson's ds / Cerebellar ds, Wilson's ds, Alcohol, MS

P / C W A M

DDx: *"I'd like to ask you a few questions to rule out other causes."*

Resting Tremor (Parkinsons Disease) — *"Do you have a tremor when you are resting? Is it like a pin-rolling tremor?*

Intentional Tremor (Cerebellar, Wilson's Disease, Alcohol, MS) — *"Do you get tremors when you are about to do something or some action? Do you drink alcohol? How often? Are you on any medications? Do you have any hx of heart conditions? Any hx of stroke in the past? Do you have any f/hx of a condition related to copper in the body or past med hx with that? Are you on any medication? Do you have relapses of any situations which involve difficulty walking/ vision /or issues with bladder control?"*

Name / Age

PC - Empathy

SOCRATES——------------------Impact

b/b

N.W.T.

BE FAST

DDx At Rest: P

Intention: C W A M

Postural: ETG P a d d LK

Neuro Hx — HV LWN BCSSS - SAM

P A M H U G S F O S S

|

S A D - COCAINE

Tremors (Continued)

Postural tremor:

Essential Thyroid Glucose Panic Attack Diet Drugs CLD CKD

E T G Pa d d L K

<u>Postural Tremors</u> (Essential tremors, Thyroid, Glucose, Panic attack, Diet, Drugs, Chronic Liver Disease, Chronic Kidney Disease) — "*Do you have any hx of diabetes? Are you on any medication for that? Do you feel thirsty a lot? Do you pee a lot? Do you feel cold when others do not? Are you the type of person who is anxious a lot or has had panic attacks in the past? How about your diet? Do you take enough vitamins? Are you someone who drinks a lot of coffee? Are you on any medications? Any hx of chronic liver disease or chronic kidney disease?*"

Name / Age

PC - Empathy

SOCRATES——------------------Impact

b/b

N.W.T.

BE FAST

SIGN POST

DDx At Rest: P

Intention: C W A M

Postural: ETG P a d d LK

Neuro Hx — HV LWN BCSSS - SAM

P A M H U G S F O S S

|

S A D - COCAINE

Parkinson's Disease

Pt comes with TRAP

"Just to make sure there's nothing serious going on."

b/b — *"Any bladder and bowel changes?"*

NWT — *"Any numbness, weakness or tingling of any part of your body?"*

BE FAST — Qs to rule out stroke (Refer to Key)

Tremors Rigidity Akinesia Postural Instability

T R A P

DDx: *"I'd like to ask you a few questions to rule out other causes."*

Tremor — *"Do you have a tremor when you are resting? Is it like a pin-rolling tremor?"*

Rigidity — *"Do you find you have stiffness or rigidity when you move your arms or legs? Have you noticed if you have any jerky slow movements?"*

Akinesia — *"Have you noticed a loss of arm swing while walking? Difficulty initiating movement? Slow to think?"*

Postural Instability — Stooped posture, shuffling gait.

Name / Age

PC - Empathy

SOCRATES——————————Impact

b/b

N.W.T.

BE FAST

DDx T R A P

Neuro Hx — HV LWN BCSSS - SAM

Psych Hx — MOAPS – C

ADLs/IADLs

P A M H U G S F O S S

|

S A D

Dizziness/Vertigo

SOCRATES – Clarify if it is:

Vertigo — *"When you say dizziness do you mean that the room is spinning?"*

Syncope — *"Or do you feel lightheaded and faint?"*

Cerebellar ataxia — *"Do you notice difficulty in walking & is putting you off balance?"*

Vertigo – Central (Constant)

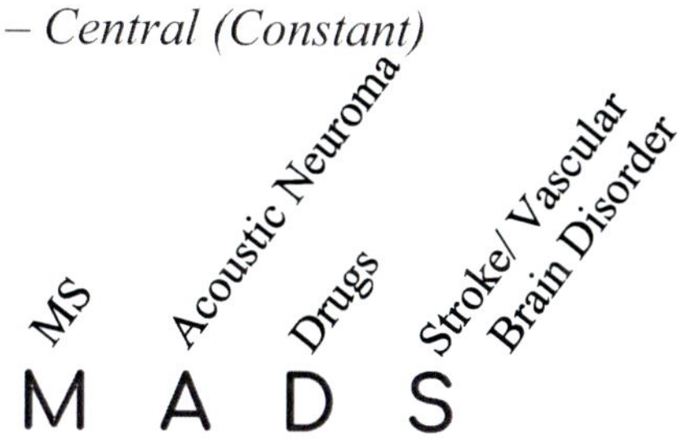

SIGN POST DDx: *"I'd like to ask you a few questions to rule out other causes."*

Multiple Sclerosis (MS) — Chronic relapsing (previous episodes), NWT, b/b vision/gait/speech issues, loss of balance, falls, also depression.

Acoustic Neuroma — Unilateral HL/ Weight loss.

Drugs — PCP, Aspirin, blood thinners, alcohol.

Stroke/ Vascular Brain Disorder — **NWT**, **BE FAST**. hx of HTN/ heart disease.

VERTIGO — *"For how long has it been going on?"*

Name / Age

PC - Empathy

SOCRATES--------------------**Impact**

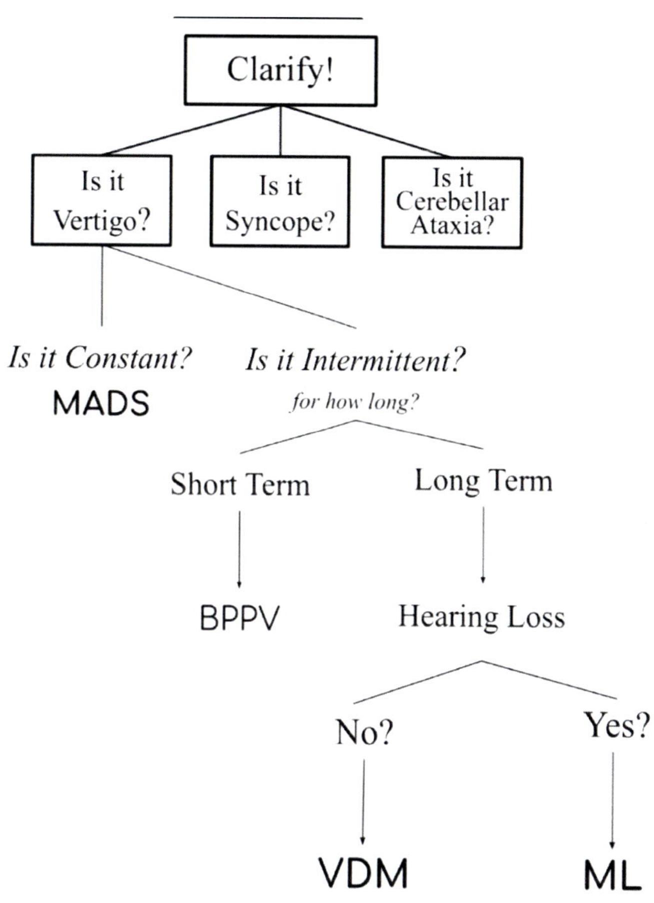

Neuro Hx — HV LWN BCSSS - SAM

P A M H U G S F O S S

|

S A D

Dizziness/Vertigo (Continued)

Vertigo intermittent — (Short time)
BPPV — Benign Paroxysmal positional vertigo.

Vertigo - Intermittent - (long time) – Ask about Hearing Loss — if NO:

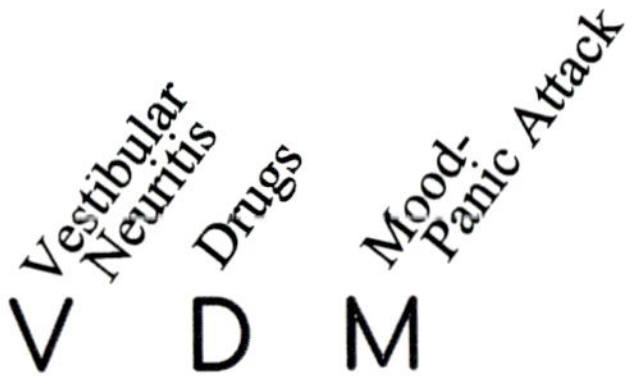

SIGN POST DDx: *"I'd like to ask you a few questions to rule out other causes."*

Vestibular Neuritis — *"Did you find that you are veering to one side when walking? Any Ear d/c?"*
Drugs — *"Are you on any medications?"*
Mood- Panic Attack — *"Are you the type of person who is anxious a lot or has had panic attacks in the past?"* Ask about symptoms of panic attacks.

Vertigo - Intermittent - (long time) – Ask about Hearing Loss — If YES:

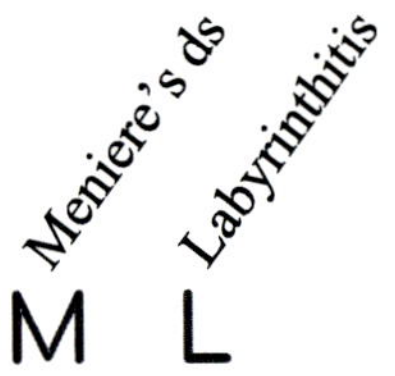

Labyrinthitis — *"Any prior flu-like symptoms? Any prior ear infections?"*
Meniere's disease — *"Have you experienced any ringing in your ears? Or a feeling of fullness in your ear?"*

Name / Age

PC - Empathy

SOCRATES--------------------**Impact**

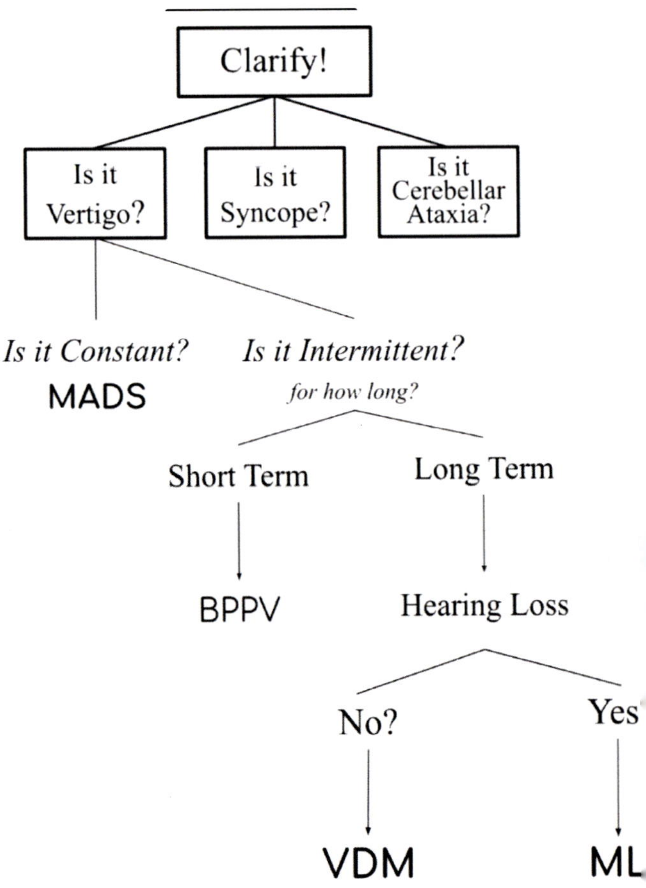

Neuro Hx — HV LWN BCSSS - SAM

P A M H U G S F O S S

S A D

Gait

Pt has difficulty walking and/or hx of falls

🚩 b/b — *"Any bladder and bowel changes?"*

NWT — *"Any numbness, weakness or tingling of any part of your body?"*

BE FAST — Qs to rule out stroke (Refer to Key)

MS, Cerebellar ds, Vestibular ds, Radiculopathy, Stroke, Parkinson's disease, Eye, P. Neuropathy, Dementia/ Delirium, Alcohol, NPH, Trauma

Ms CVR'S PENDANT

Jt /GBS

SIGN POST DDx: *"I'd like to ask you a few questions to rule out other causes."*

Multiple Sclerosis (MS) — Chronic relapsing (previous episodes), NWT, b/b vision/gait/speech issues, loss of balance, falls, also depression.

Cerebellar Stroke/ Lesion — *"Any difficulty with Speech or swallowing? Any involuntary eye movements?"* (nystagmus)

Vestibular — *"Any ear d/c? hearing loss? Vertigo? Do you find that you are veering/deviating to one side when walking?"*

Radiculopathy — *"Any associated Pain radiating to the leg or buttocks?"*

Stroke — **BE FAST**

Parkinsons — TRAP. Shuffling gait. Difficult to initiate movement.

Name / Age

PC - Empathy

SOCRATES——--------------------**Impact**

🚩 b/b

N.W.T.

BE FAST

SIGN POST DDx

Ms CVR's PENDANT

Jt/GBS

Neuro Hx — HV LWN BCSSS - SAM

P A M H U G S F O S S

|

S A D

Gait (Continued)

MS Cerebellar ds Vestibular ds Radiculopathy Stroke Parkinson's disease Eye P. Neuropathy Dementia/ Delirium Alcohol NPH Trauma

Ms CVR'S PENDANT

Jt /GBS

<u>Parkinson's disease</u> — Ask TRAP (Refer to Parkinson's disease)

<u>Eye</u> — *"Has your vision declined? Do you find it difficult to read the ticker on TV or drive? Any difficulty reading?"*

<u>Peripheral Neuropathy</u> — DM/ B12- *"Any associated tingling or pins and needles sensation on your arm or leg?"* Ask about diet and vitamin supplements.

<u>Dementia/ Delirium</u> — *"Have you noticed any decline in your memory? Notice any confusion? Any recent hospitalization or surgery?"*

<u>Alcohol</u> — *"Do you drink alcohol? How often?"*

<u>Normal pressure Hydrocephalus</u> — *"Any associated urinary incontinence?/memory decline or confusion?"*

<u>Trauma /Rheumatology /Guillain-Barre Syndrome (GBS)</u> — *"Any hx of trauma? Any morning stiffness or joint pain? Are the symptoms appearing in an ascending fashion? Did you have a recent diarrheal episode?"*

Name / Age

PC - Empathy

SOCRATES---------------------**Impact**

b/b

N.W.T.

BE FAST

SIGN POST DDx

Ms CVR's PENDANT

Jt/GBS

Neuro Hx — HV LWN BCSSS - SAM

P A M H U G S F O S S

|

S A D

Concussions

SIGN POST — *"Just to make sure there's nothing serious going on."*

F (Fracture of basal skull) A (Amnesia) G (↓ GCS) V (persistent Vomiting)

Basal skull fracture — *"Have you noticed any d/c from your ears or nose? Any bruising around your eyes or back of ears?"*

- Ask detailed hx of the trauma event.
- Ask about s/s for concussion- Confusion, delayed response, emotional changes, headache, pain, dizziness, amnesia, loss of consciousness, raised ICP.
- This would most probably be a counselling station.

Name / Age

PC - Empathy

SOCRATES—-------------------Impact

Trauma

F A G V

Neuro Hx — HV LWN BCSSS - SAM

P A M H U G S F O S S

S A D (from S of HUGS)

Seizures

SOCRATES — *Before? During? After?*

Clarify if it was a seizure or syncope.

"What were you doing before the episode? Were you with someone when it happened? Was your whole body having jerky movements or only one leg or arm? Did you bite your tongue? Did you pee yourself? How were you doing after? Any drowsiness? Did you hit your head or hurt yourself? Any memory loss?'

"Just to make sure there's nothing serious going on."

Stroke Trauma Fever Infection Tumor Sleep/ Stress Withdrawal Epilepsy Electrolytes Drugs

St Fits Weed

DDx: *"I'd like to ask you a few questions to rule out other causes."*

Stoke — **BE FAST**

Trauma — *"Did you hurt yourself?*

Fever/Infection – Meningitis/ Encephalitis — *"Any fever? Neck stiffness? Chills? Nausea/vomiting? Confusion? LOC? Any rashes?"*

Tumor — *"Any weight loss? night sweats/fever? Hx of cancer or f/hx of cancer?"*

Sleep/ Stress — *"How is your sleep hygiene? Any recent stressors in life?"*

Name / Age

PC - Empathy

SOCRATES--------------------**Impact**

Before? During? After?

Trauma

Fever, neck stiffness

Prolonged post-ictal phase.

Focal neural deficit

DDx **St Fits Weed**

Neuro Hx — HV LWN BCSSS - SAM

P A M H U G S F O S S

S A D

Seizures (Continued)

Stroke Trauma Fever Infection Tumor Sleep/ Stress Withdrawal Epilepsy Electrolytes Drugs

St Fits Weed

Withdrawal — Ask about alcohol and drug intake (Lithium, cocaine)

Epilepsy — *"Any hx of epilepsy or previous episodes of seizures?"*

Electrolytes — Hypoglycemia/ Hypocalcemia. *"Are you a diabetic? Did you take your insulin or change the dose? How was your diet that day? Were you feeling hungry? Did you notice any tremors or shakiness before the seizure? Did you notice any tingling sensation around the mouth? Any painful spasms of hands or feet?"*

Name / Age

PC - Empathy

SOCRATES--------------------**Impact**

Before? During? After?

Trauma

Fever, neck stiffness

Prolonged post-ictal phase.

Focal neural deficit

DDx **St Fits Weed**

Neuro Hx — HV LWN BCSSS - SAM

P A M H U G S F O S S

S A D

Stroke

"Just to make sure there's nothing serious going on."

MS Psychosis P. Neuropathy TIA Space occupying lesion Cervical Radiculopathy

Ms P N T S cr

DDx: *"I'd like to ask you a few questions to rule out other causes."*

Multiple Sclerosis (MS) — Chronic relapsing (previous episodes), NWT, b/b vision/gait/speech issues, loss of balance, falls, also depression.

Psychosis — *"Are you being treated for any mental illness?"*

P. Neuropathy — NWT

TIA (Reversible) — *"Have you had similar symptoms that resolved quickly? Did your symptoms completely disappear?"*

Space Occupying Lesion — *"Have you noticed any severe headaches? Blurry vision or loss of vision? Any hx of tumors in the body? Any f/hx of cancer? Any weight loss/night sweats/fever?"*

Cervical Radiculopathy — "Any associated pain shooting down your leg or buttocks?"

Name / Age

PC - Empathy

SOCRATES——------------------**Impact**

b/b

N.W.T.

BE FAST

DDx **Ms PNTS cr**

Neuro Hx — HV LWN BCSSS - SAM

P A M   H U G S   F O S S

|

S A D

Subarachnoid Hemorrhage

SOCRATES – Acute, worst headache ever, worse on exertion.

SIGN POST *"Just to make sure there's nothing serious going on."*

- **D** – neural Deficits
- **a** – upon Awakening
- **f** – Fever
- **t** – Thunderclap headache
- **n** – New Headache, Neck Stiffness
- **e** – on Exertion
- **s** – Scalp Tenderness
- **s** – Seizures

D a f t n e s s

RF:

- **H** – HTN
- **A** – Aneurysms
- **P** – Pregnancy
- **O** – OCP
- **S** – Smoking
- **A** – Alcohol
- **D** – Drugs

HAPO SAD

SIGN POST RF: *"I'd like to ask you a few questions to rule out any risk factors."*

"Do you have any hx of high blood pressure?"

Can ask about associated conditions with aneurysms e.g, Polycystic kidney disease, fibromuscular ds, f/hx of aneurysms, (Ehler Danlos/ Marfan's/ Osler's), HTN, trauma, endometrial cancer. *"Are you pregnant by any chance? Are you on any oral contraceptive pills?"* Ask about **SAD**.

Name / Age

PC - Empathy

SOCRATES—-------------------**Impact**

Trauma!

D a f t n e s s

RF: HAPO SAD

Neuro Hx — HV LWN BCSSS - SAM

P A M H U G S F O S S

|

S A D — COCAINE

Sleep Apnea

Pt is tired and may present with morning headaches. BP 140/90

SIGN POST *"Just to make sure there's nothing serious going on."*

GERD COPD Depression Insomnia Cardiac Tonsils Asthma Thyroid Opioid User Restless Leg syndrome

G C D I C T A T O R

SIGN POST DDx: *"I'd like to ask you a few questions to rule out other causes."*

<u>GERD</u> — *"Any chest pain after meals? Any hx of heartburn/sour taste in mouth/chronic cough?"*

<u>COPD</u> — *"Any hx of chronic cough or **SOB**?"*

<u>Depression</u> — *"How is your mood been lately? Are you feeling depressed/decreased concentration/ feelings of guilt? Have you thought of hurting yourself?"*

<u>Insomnia</u> — *"Do you have difficulty falling asleep or staying asleep? How is your sleep hygiene?"*

<u>Cardiac</u> — *"Any hx of heart conditions?"*

<u>Tonsils</u> — *"Has anyone noticed that you snore or have noisy breathing while sleeping?"*

<u>Asthma</u> — *"Do you have shortness of breath? Any allergies? Do you use an inhaler? Family hx of asthma?"*

Name / Age

PC - Empathy

SOCRATES------------------------**Impact**

If high blood pressure ask for **CHUDS** (Refer to HTN)

SIGN POST DDx **GC DICTATOR**

RF: **S T O P B A N G**

Can also ask complications: **C S H A P E D**

Neuro Hx — HV LWN BCSSS - SAM

P A M H U G S F O S S

|

S A D

Sleep Apnea (Continued)

GERD, COPD, Depression, Insomnia, Cardiac, Tonsils, Asthma, Thyroid, Opioid User, Restless Leg syndrome

G C D I C T A T O R

DDx: *"I'd like to ask you a few questions to rule out other causes."*

Thyroid — *"Any issues with your thyroid in the past? Do you feel hot or cold when others don't?"*

Opioid User — *"Have you ever tried recreational drugs? Do you use opioids? How often?"*

Restless Leg Syndrome — *"Do you feel the urge to move or shake your leg when resting or at bedtime? Have you ever been diagnosed with iron deficiency?"*

Snoring, Tiredness, observed Apnea, high blood Pressure, BMI - ↑35, Age - ↑50, Neck circumference, Gender (Male)

RF: **S T O P B A N G**

Complications of sleep apnea can be:

Cardiac Ds, Stroke, HTN, motor vehicle Accident, Polycythemia, Erectile Dysfunction, DM

C S H A P E D

Name / Age

PC - Empathy

SOCRATES———————————**Impact**

If high blood pressure ask for **CHUDS** (Refer to HTN)

DDx **GC DICTATOR**

RF: **S T O P B A N G**

Can also ask complications: **C S H A P E D**

Neuro Hx — HV LWN BCSSS - SAM

P A M H U G S F O S S

S A D

Facial Palsy

MS
Bell's Palsy
Ramsay Hunt syndrome
Infections
Stroke
Tumor/ Trauma
Malignant Otitis Externa
Lyme ds
Sarcoidosis
GBS

Ms. B R I S T O L S. G

SIGN POST DDx: *"I'd like to ask you a few questions to rule out other causes."*

<u>Multiple sclerosis</u> — Chronic relapsing (previous episodes), NWT, b/b vision/gait/speech issues, loss of balance, falls, also depression.

<u>Bell's palsy</u> — Acute onset, numbness of the ear, ↑sensitivity to sound, no hearing loss.

<u>Ramsay Hunt Syndrome</u> — Acute onset, vesicles on the ear. PAINFUL, on the ear/ face/ mouth/ sensorineural hearing loss/ ↑Sensitivity to sound.

<u>Infections</u> — (Syphilis, TB, Mumps, Meningitis, EBV) — *"Travel hx, sick contact, sexual hx, neck stiffness, b/w facial swelling, painful balls."*

<u>Stroke</u> — **BE FAST**. If middle cerebral artery – numbness /weakness of the arm. If anterior inferior cerebellar artery – difficulty swallowing, speaking, ↓vision, double vision, hearing loss, difficulty balancing and walking.

Name / Age

PC - Empathy

SOCRATES——------------------**Impact**

SIGN POST DDx **Ms. BRISTOLS. G**

Neuro Hx — HV LWN BCSSS - SAM

P A M H U G S F O S S

|

S A D

Facial Palsy (Continued)

MS, Bell's Palsy, Ramsay Hunt syndrome, Infections, Stroke, Tumor/ Trauma, Malignant Otitis Externa, Lyme ds, Sarcoidosis, GBS

Ms. B R I S T O L S. G

<u>Trauma/ Tumor</u> — at the cerebellar Pontine angle. *"Any hx of trauma? Any weight loss/ night sweats/ fever? Any hx of cancer or f/hx of cancer?"*

<u>Malignant Otitis Externa</u> (MOE) — Pt can be elderly with DM or immunocompromised, ear pain, yellowish ear d/c, and may have CN involved (CN10 & CN11).

<u>Lyme disease</u> — Travel hx/ camping hx. *"Any hx of a rash? or tick bite?"*

<u>Sarcoidosis</u> — *"Do you have a hx of chronic cough? Have you noticed any painful red lesions on your legs?"*

<u>Guillain-Barre Syndrome (GBS)</u> — *"Any hx of diarrhea? Have you noticed any acute paralysis starting from your legs upwards?"*

Name / Age

PC - Empathy

SOCRATES——————————**Impact**

SIGN POST DDx **Ms. BRISTOLS. G**

Neuro Hx — HV LWN BCSSS - SAM

P A M   H U G S   F O S S

S A D

Hoarseness

SOCRATES — *"Any associated fever, pain, difficulty swallowing, swelling of the neck, change in voice, hirsutism? Any cough, repeated infections, or* ***SOB****?"*

Laryngitis Pharyngitis laryngeal CA vocal Polyps Papillomatosis vocal Nodule Thyroid MS GERD Stroke

L PC Po Pa NoT Ms GS

SIGN POST DDx: *"I'd like to ask you a few questions to rule out other causes."*

<u>Laryngitis/Pharyngitis</u> — Prior hx of throat infection/ viral infection, toxic fume inhalation, repeated infections, chronic change in voice, hx of postnasal drip/GERD, hx of voice strain *"Any activity you do that requires repeated use of voice?"*

<u>Laryngeal tumor</u> — *"Any hx of trauma? Any weight loss/night sweats/fever? Any hx of cancer or f/hx of cancer?"*

<u>Vocal Polyps</u> — Pt would be a 30-50 yr old male, hx of smoking, allergies or GERD. Symptoms of voice change, +/- dyspnea aphonia, cough attacks and voice strain.

Name / Age

PC - Empathy

SOCRATES-------------------**Impact**

SIGN POST DDx

L PC PoPa NoT Ms GS

Neuro Hx — HV LWN BCSSS - SAM

P A M   H U G S   F O S S

|

S A D

Hoarseness (Continued)

Laryngitis, Pharyngitis, laryngeal CA, vocal Polyps, Papillomatosis, vocal Nodule, Thyroid, MS, GERD, Stroke

L PC Po Pa NoT Ms GS

Benign Laryngeal Papillomatosis— Child with hx of stridor, repeated pneumonia, hemoptysis, dysphagia, FTT, wheezing or chronic cough.

Vocal Nodule — *"Do you have to use your voice a lot at work? Is it worse end of day?"* Jobs include: singer, school teacher, bartender, works with children, etc.

Thyroid — *"Any issues with your thyroid in the past? Do you feel hot or cold when others don't?"*

Multiple Sclerosis — Chronic relapsing (previous episodes), NWT, b/b vision/gait/speech issues, loss of balance, falls, also depression.

GERD — *"Any chest pain after meals? Any hx of heartburn/sour taste in mouth/chronic cough?"*

Stroke — **BE FAST.**

Name / Age

PC - Empathy

SOCRATES--------------------**Impact**

SIGN POST DDx

L PC PoPa NoT Ms GS

Neuro Hx — HV LWN BCSSS - SAM

P A M   H U G S   F O S S

S A D

Multiple Sclerosis

"Just to make sure there's nothing serious going on."

Multiple Sclerosis, Psychosis, P. Neuropathy, TIA, Space occupying lesion, Cervical Radiculopathy

Ms P N T S cr

DDx: *"I'd like to ask you a few questions to rule out other causes."*

Refer to Stroke.

<u>S/s of Multiple Sclerosis-</u>

Weakness, Ataxia, Tremors/Toilet issues, Speech/Swallow, Optic Neuritis, Nystagmus, ↑ s/s in Heat, Electrical sensation

W A T S O N HE

<u>S/S</u> — *"Any weakness/ numbness in any part of your body? Do you have any difficulty walking? Have you noticed any accidents with your bladder? Any difficulty talking or swallowing? Are you experiencing any double vision? Any blurry vision or pain in eye movement? And do these symptoms worsen in heat? Any electrical sensations in the neck on neck flexion?"*

Name / Age

PC - Empathy

SOCRATES——-----------------Impact

b/b

N.W.T.

BE FAST

DDx **Ms PNTS cr**

S/S **- W A T S O N HE**

Neuro Hx — HV LWN BCSSS - SAM

P A M H U G S F O S S

P A M ↓ Sarcoidosis

F O S S ↓ of MS/SLE

Psychiatry

How to organise yourself before entering the station + KEY **226**

Panic Attack **232**

Depression **233**

OCD **234**

Mania **236**

Schizophrenia **237**

Anorexia Nervosa **238**

Dementia **240**

Delirium **242**

Suicide **244**

Insomnia **244**

Fatigue **245**

How to organise yourself before entering the station

Before entering the station, you will have under two minutes to read the prompt and jot down notes in your booklet.

These notes should focus on key information you'll need to remember while taking the history from the standardized participant (SP). The SP is an actor trained to portray a specific medical condition or scenario. Their purpose is to interact with you and allow the physician examiner (PE) to observe and assess your performance.

The booklet provided is rectangular, about half the size of an A4 sheet. It contains blank sheets for your notes, as well as candidate code stickers, which you'll need to hand over to the examiner before starting each station.

Given the time constraints and anxiety during the station, these notes can serve as a valuable guide to help you complete a thorough history.

Therefore, it is essential to practice responding to prompts and mastering the '2-minute drill' regularly to achieve your best results.

HOW TO PRACTICE :

For practice purposes, folding an A4 sheet in half works well to simulate the booklet.

Hence this book is divided into two columns:

Left column	**Right column**
Contains a breakdown of the mnemonics and the questions you may need to ask.	Notes to write in your booklet as part of your 2-minute drill, often including mnemonics that make the best use of your time and help you recall essential steps efficiently!

These structured notes will provide a clear and concise roadmap to ensure you stay focused and efficient during the station.

The KEY

Knock on the door, Walk in, Wear a smile, Greet the examiner, and hand the candidate code, *"Hi, here's my candidate code."*
Sanitize your hands and simultaneously:

Introduce yourself to the standardized participant (SP):
"Hello, I am Dr___ and I will be your physician today. May I know your name and age, please? How would you like to be addressed? That's great!

"Is it okay if I sit down and take a few notes?"

PC: Presenting Complaints
"What brings you in here today?"
Listen to the patient. It is important to express **Empathy.**
"I am sorry to hear that. That must be quite distressing."

"Okay, so I would like to ask you a few questions and do a physical exam after, and we will figure out a treatment plan for you today!"

SOCRATES-B: For conditions with other symptoms, SOCRATES-B can still be used.

- site: *"Where is the pain? Can you point at it?"*
- onset: *"Was it gradual or sudden in onset?"*
- character: *"What kind of pain is it? Is it a dull pain or a sharp pain?"*
- radiate: *"Does the pain radiate anywhere?"*
- associated symptoms: *"Any associated symptoms?"*
- time: *"Is the pain constant or intermittent?"*
- exacerbating factor: *"Does anything relieve the pain or make it worse?"*
- severity: *"On a scale from 1-10, how would you rate the pain? 10 being the worst."*
- before: *"Have you had this before?"*

Not every P/C involves pain. Some complaints may just require 'o-ate' onset associated s/s, time, and exacerbating/ relieving factors.

COCA-b: For any vomiting/discharge/sputum/stool/urine.
Colour, **O**dor, **C**onsistency, **A**mount, **B**lood (If yes for blood, ask **BBL**)

BBL — (if pt complains of bleeding), stands for :

- <u>B</u>lood thinners – *"Are you on blood thinners?"*
- <u>B</u>loody Diarrhea – *"Do you bruise easily or bleed easily?"*
- <u>L</u>iver Disease — *"Any hx of liver disease?"*

Impact: *"How are you coping with this?"*

DDX: Differentials for the condition given for each condition.

SIGNPOST: This symbol means you have to signpost! A signpost is an introductory statement. This is to introduce your segment of questions so the examiner is aware of your line of questioning.

E.g.: DDx - means you have to place an introductory statement before asking for differentials: *"I am going to ask a few questions to rule out any other causes."*

Red flags: This is for conditions we need to rule out right away as they may require urgent attention.

PAM HUGS FOSS: stands for:

- Past medical hx: *"Since this is the first time we are meeting, do you have any past medical conditions that I should know about? Or that you have been treated for?"*
- Allergies: *"Do you have any allergies?"*
- Medications: *"Are you on any medications? What are the medications? Are you adherent with your medications? What is the dosage?"*
- Hospitalization/Surgery: *"Have you ever been hospitalized before? Any surgeries done before?"*
- Urinary changes: *"Have you noticed changes in your urine?"*
- GIT changes: *"Have you noticed any changes in your bowel habits?"*
- SAD- **S**moking/**A**lcohol/Recreational **D**rugs:
    - *"Do you smoke? How many cigarettes a day? For how long? Have you ever thought about quitting?"*
    - *"Do you drink alcohol? How often?"*
    - *"Have you done any recreational drugs? What have you used? How do you take it? Do you sniff or inject? Do you share needles?"*
- Family history: *"Any family history of any medical conditions?"* Specific medical conditions you are concerned about.
- Occupation: *"If I may ask, what do you do for a living?"*
- Social: *"May I know about your living conditions? Who do you live with?"*
- Support: *"Do you have any family around? Are they supportive? That's good to know."*

Mnemonics for system questions:
Psych:
MOoAPS – C

- Mood — *"How has your mood been? Are you uninterested in the things you previously enjoyed? And how about the opposite? Do you ever get a high mood and energy? Have you had any previous diagnosis?"*
- Organic illness (Other differentials) — *"Just to make sure you don't have anything else going on...."*
- OCD — *"Are you the type of person who checks on things again and again? Do you ever have any compulsive thoughts that you want to act on?"*
- Anxiety — *"Are you the type of person who worries a lot?"* If yes: Ask (C FIRST) about decreased Concentration, Fatigue, irritability, sleep issues, and muscle tension. *"Do you sometimes get panic attacks? [What is a panic attack? " Sometimes when people have spells of anxiety they may experience shortness of breath, heart racing and sweating. Is that something you have?"]*
- Psychosis — *"I would like to ask a few more standard questions. Do you see or hear things that other people don't? Do you have any thoughts that somebody is keeping a tab on you or putting thoughts in your head? Do you feel that you have special powers? Do you often think somebody's following you?"*
- Suicidal or homicidal Ideation — *"Do you have any thoughts of harming yourself? or somebody else?"*
- Collateral hx — *"Is it ok if I speak to your mom [or guardian], just to get a collateral hx?"*

MBUSS - additional history taking for elderly patients

- Memory changes
- Bowel habits
- Urinary changes
- Sleep changes
- Support system— *"Tell me a little about your living situation. Any family members nearby?"*

FOR PANIC ATTACK- **Psst Nd 3Cs**

- Palpitations
- Shaking/ trembling
- Shortness of Breath
- Nausea
- Depersonalization/ Derealization
- Feeling of being out of Control
- Choking or sensation of dying
- Chest pain

CRITERIA FOR DEPRESSION (≥ 5 for 2 weeks)-- **G CAT WAS SAD** -

- Guilty - *" Do you find yourself feeling a sense of guilt?"*
- Concentration — *"Do you find you have decreased concentration lately?"*
- Anhedonia — *"Do you feel you have lost interest in things you were interested in before?"*
- Tiredness/Fatigue — *"Do you feel tired most of the time?"*
- Weight loss — *"Have you lost any weight?"*
- Appetite — *"How is your appetite? Are you eating properly?"*
- Sleep — *"How about your sleep?"*
- Suicide — *"Have you ever thought that you'd be better off dead? Have you tried to harm/kill yourself?"*
    - If YES → Jump to **SAD PERSONS** (screening)
- Agitation — *"Do you find yourself agitated a lot?"*
- Depression — *"How is your mood these days?"*

CRITERIA FOR MANIA (≥ 3 for 1 week)-**GST PAID**

- Grandiosity — *"Do you feel you have special powers or a unique purpose?"*
- Sleep (decreased need) — *"How's your sleep?"*
- Talkative — *"You seem to be talking fast, do you feel like you are having a flight of ideas?"*
- Pleasurable Activities, Painful Consequences — *"Have you done anything unusual that you wouldn't normally do, like taking risks that you wouldn't normally take? Have you spent a lot of money on anything lately?"*
- Activity (Increased) — *"What have you been doing lately?"*
- Ideas (flight of) — *"You seem to be talking fast, do you feel like you are having a flight of ideas?"*
- Distractible — *"Do you find that you are distracted easily?"*

FOR ANXIETY **- C FIRST**

- Concentration
- Fatigue
- Irritability
- Restlessness
- Stress
- muscle Tension

SAD PERSONS (Suicide Screening)

- Sex — Male sex
- Age (<19 or >65 years)
- Depression
- Previous attempts
- Ethanol (alcohol or substance use)
- Rational thinking loss
- Suicide in the family
- Organized plan
- No support system
- Sickness/Serious illness

Panic Attack

SOCRATES + **Psst Nd 3Cs** - for Panic attack

"Just to make sure there's nothing serious going on."

Thyroid Glucose Anemia Pheochromocytoma

T G A P

DDx: *"I'd like to ask you a few questions to rule out other causes."*

<u>Thyroid</u> — *"Do you feel hot or sweaty when others don't? Have you noticed recent weight loss despite having a good appetite?"*

<u>Glucose</u> — *"Have you eaten anything today? When was your last meal?"*

<u>Anemia</u> — *"Do you find that you are paler than everyone else? Any hx of blood disorders? Do you bleed easily or bruise easily?"*

<u>Pheochromocytoma</u> — *"Any hx of pulsating headaches? Any perspiration associated with the heart racing?"*

Name / Age

PC - Empathy

SOCRATES---------------------**Impact**

\+ **Psst Nd 3Cs** - for Panic attack

Hx of heart disease

Hx of MI

DDx T G A P

↑

Other causes

↑

Psych Hx- MOoAPS

P A M H U G S F O S S

|

S A D

Depression

SOCRATES + **G CAT WAS SAD** - criteria for depression (≥ 5 for 2 weeks) + MOoAPS Hx

Thyroid Anemia Medications Alcohol Drugs

T A Med A D

DDx: *"I'd like to ask you a few questions to rule out other causes."*

Thyroid — *"Have you had any thyroid issues in the past? Do you have any heat or cold tolerance?"*

Anemia — *"Do you find that you are paler than everyone else? Any hx of blood disorders? Do you bleed easily or bruise easily?"*

Medications — *"Are there any medications you take? Dosage/duration?"*

Alcohol — *"Do you drink alcohol? How often do you drink alcohol?"*

Drugs — *"Have you done any recreational drugs? What have you used? How do you take it? Do you sniff or inject? Do you share needles?"*

Name / Age

PC - Empathy

SOCRATES——------------------Impact

\+ **'G CAT WAS SAD'** -criteria for depression (≥ 5 for 2 weeks)

DDx TAMed AD

↑

Other causes

↑

Psych Hx- MOoAPS

Suicide screening -

SAD PERSONS (≥ 5 - Hospitalize)

P A M H U G S F O S S

|

S A D

OCD

SOCRATES + **MOoAPS Hx** + OCD qs:
"Are you the type of person who checks things again and again? What makes you do that? Ok, so there are thoughts that come into your mind? How does that make you feel? Do you find them intrusive? Have you tried to resist?
Do you need things to be in a particular order? If not, do you get distressed? What do you do to relieve the stress/anxiety/ thoughts? Does it make you feel less anxious? What would happen if you performed the action? Does it affect your work/relationship?"

PTSD, Hypochondriasis, Autism, Tic ds, Body Dysmorphia, Eating ds, Trichotillomania

P H A T B E T

DDx: *"I'd like to ask you a few questions to rule out other causes."*

PTSD — *"Do your intrusive thoughts seem directly related to a specific traumatic event you've experienced?"*
Hypochondriasis — *"Are you preoccupied with a fear of serious illness? Do you find yourself repeatedly seeking medical reassurance?"*
Autism — *"Do you struggle with social interactions or communication skills?"*
Tic disorder — *"Do you experience sudden repetitive movements or make sounds that are out of your control?"*

Name / Age

PC - Empathy

SOCRATES—-------------------Impact

+ **OCD qs.**

DDx P H A T B E T

↑

Other causes

↑

Psych Hx- MOoAPS

P A M H U G S F O S S

|

S A D

OCD (Continued)

PTSD, Hypochondriasis, Autism, Tic ds — Body Dysmorphia, Eating ds, Trichotillomania

P H A T B E T

Body dysmorphia — *"Are you excessively concerned by your appearance and find yourself frequently checking or trying to fix it?"*

Eating disorder — *"Are you preoccupied with thoughts about your weight? Do you have a fear of eating?"*

Trichotillomania — *"Do you feel an urge to pull out your hair? Does this bring you relief or satisfaction?"*

Name / Age

PC - Empathy

SOCRATES——------------------Impact

\+ **OCD qs.**

DDx **P H A T B E T**

↑

Other causes

↑

Psych Hx- MOoAPS

P A M H U G S F O S S

|

S A D

Mania

SOCRATES + **GST PAID**- criteria for mania (≥ 3 for 1 week) + **MOoAPS Hx**

"Just to make sure there's nothing serious going on."

Lithium, Infection, Thyroid, Trauma, Alcohol, Drug

L i T T A D

DDx: *"I'd like to ask you a few questions to rule out other causes."*

Lithium — *"Have you noticed any changes in your vision? Any blurriness? Any difficulty seeing in your periphery? Have you experienced any headaches? Any weight gain? Any nipple discharge?"*

Infection — *"Do you have a fever? Any hx of sick contacts? Any hx of travel?"*

Thyroid — *"Do you feel hot or sweaty when others don't? Have you noticed recent weight loss despite having a good appetite?"*

Trauma — *"Any hx of trauma?"*

Alcohol — *"Do you drink alcohol? How often? How many glasses a day?"*

Drugs — *"Have you done any recreational drugs? What have you used? How do you take it?"*

Name / Age

PC - Empathy

SOCRATES--------------------Impact

+ **GST PAID** for mania (≥ 3 for 1 week)

No support

Suicidical

Substance abuse

DDx LiTT AD

↑

Other causes

↑

Psych Hx- MOoAPS

P A M H U G S F O S S

|

S A D

Schizophrenia

SOCRATES + MOoAPS Hx

"Just to make sure there's nothing serious going on."

Thyroid Infection Medication Substance abuse

T i Me S

DDx: *"I'd like to ask you a few questions to rule out other causes."*

<u>Thyroid</u> — *"Do you feel hot or sweaty when others don't? Have you noticed recent weight loss despite having a good appetite?"*

<u>Infection</u> — *"Do you have a fever? Any hx of sick contacts? Any hx of travel?"*

<u>Medication</u> — *"Are there any medications you take? Dosage/duration?"*

<u>Substance Abuse</u> — *"Have you done any recreational drugs? What have you used? How do you take it?"*

Name / Age

PC - Empathy

SOCRATES--------------------**Impact**

No support

Suicidical

Substance abuse

DDx **T i Me s**

↑

Other causes

↑

Psych Hx- MOoAPS

P A M   H U G S   F O S S

|

S A D

Anorexia Nervosa

SOCRATES + Eating disorder qs:

Weight — *"What is your weight/ When did it start to decline? Why do you think that is?"*

Perception — *"Do you feel your current weight is appropriate for your height? Do you wear baggy clothes?"*

Diet — *"If I may ask about your diet, what do you have for breakfast? Lunch? dinner? Any snacks?"*

Exercise — *"Any activities or sports that you do?How often"*

Extra measures — *"Have you ever tried laxatives/puking? Do you ever eat a lot and then have remorse after?"*

Impact of the eating ds — *"Have you experienced hair loss? Menstrual irregularities? Do you feel tired a lot? Bone pain? Constipation? Lightheadedness?"*

SIGN POST *"Just to make sure there's nothing serious going on."*

Diabetes Mellitus — HyperThyroidism — Tumor

D T T

SIGN POST DDx: *"I'd like to ask you a few questions to rule out other causes."*

Name / Age

PC - Empathy

SOCRATES——————————**Impact**

+ Eating ds qs

Dizzy

Faint

SIGN POST DDx D T T

↑

Other causes

↑

Psych Hx- MOoAPS

P A M H U G S F O S S

|

S A D

Anorexia Nervosa (Continued)

Diabetes Mellitus / HyperThyroidism / Tumor

D T T

Diabetes Mellitus — *"Have you noticed you have been peeing a lot? Have you been thirsty a lot? Have you been diagnosed with diabetes? Any f/hx of diabetes?"*

Hyperthyroidism — *"Do you feel hot or sweaty when others don't? Have you noticed recent weight loss despite having a good appetite?"*

Tumor — *"Any hx of cancer? Any weight loss? Any lumps or bumps on their body?"*

Name / Age

PC - Empathy

SOCRATES———————————**Impact**

+ Eating ds qs

Dizzy

Faint

SIGN POST DDx D T T

↑

Other causes

↑

Psych Hx- MOoAPS

P A M H U G S F O S S

|

S A D

Dementia

SOCRATES + **Memory assessment:** Fluctuations?/ deterioration-gradual or sudden/ Are you forgetting words/ numbers/ names/ recent events or remote events?

+ **ADLS / IADLS**

SIGN POST *"Just to make sure there's nothing serious going on."*

Degenerative, Eye/Ear, Metabolic, Emotional, Neoplastic/ NPH, Trauma, Infection, Atherosclerosis

D E M E N T I A

SIGN POST DDx: *"I'd like to ask you a few questions to rule out other causes."*

Degenerative changes (Alzheimer's, Parkinson's, Lewy body dementia) — *" Have you or your family noticed progressive memory loss that affects your daily activities?"*

Eye/Ear — *"Have you been having trouble hearing conversations? How about your vision, are you seeing clearly?"*

Metabolic — (Vitamin B12 deficiency, Wilson's disease, Uremia, Liver disease)-- - *"Have you had numbness, tingling, or balance problems along with memory issues?"*

Name / Age

PC - Empathy

SOCRATES———————————**Impact**

+ **Memory assessment**
+ **ADLS / IADLS**

Safety - *Does the pt wander off? Leave the gas on? driving?*

Substance abuse

No Support

SIGN POST DDx D E M E N T I A

↑

Other causes

↑

Psych Hx- MOoAPS

P A M   H U G S   F O S S

|

S A D

Dementia (Continued)

Degenerative, Eye/Ear, Metabolic, Emotional, Neoplastic/ NPH, Trauma, Infection, Atherosclerosis

D E M E N T I A

<u>Emotional (Pseudodementia)</u> — *"Have you been feeling sad, or hopeless? Have you lost interest in things you enjoyed doing before?"*

<u>Neoplastic</u> (Brain tumors, paraneoplastic syndromes) — *"Have you noticed any weight loss? Any night sweats? Any f/hx of cancer? Have you had any persistent headaches, vision changes, or weakness in your arms or legs?"*

<u>Trauma</u> (Chronic subdural hematoma, traumatic brain injury) — *"Have you had a hx of fall/ head injuries or repeated concussions in the past?"*

<u>Infection</u> — *"Do you have a fever? Any hx of sick contacts? Any hx of travel?"*

<u>Atherosclerosis</u> (Vascular dementia) — *"Have you had any history of stroke? Any hx of high blood pressure?"*

Name / Age

PC - Empathy

SOCRATES——------------------**Impact**

+ **Memory assessment**
+ **ADLS / IADLS**

Safety - *Does the pt wander off?*

Leave the gas on? driving?

Substance abuse

No Support

SIGN POST DDx D E M E N T I A

↑

Other causes

↑

Psych Hx- MOoAPS

P A M H U G S F O S S

S A D

Delirium

SOCRATES + Delirium questions: *"Does the patient appear to be disoriented? Are there any periods when the patient is ok? Are the symptoms Acute/ fluctuating?"*

Infection, Trauma, Sx, Medication / LETO, Stroke, Alcohol, Drugs

I t 's Me S A D

DDx: *"I'd like to ask you a few questions to rule out other causes."*

<u>Infection</u> — *"Do you have a fever? Jt pain? Teeth pain? Skin rash? Red eyes? Runny nose? Ear discharge? Sore throat? Neck stiffness? Cough? Diarrhea? Burning pee? Any hx of sick contacts? Any hx of travel?"*

<u>Trauma</u> — *"Did you hurt yourself?"* Ask about Tetanus immunization.

<u>Surgery</u> — *"Any recent hospitalization or surgeries done?"*

<u>Medications</u> — *"Are there any medications you take?Dosage/duration?" (LETO - Lithium, erythromycin, theophylline, OTC, opioids.)*

<u>Stroke</u> — N.W.T — *"Any numbness or weakness in any part of your body? Any tingling? Blurry vision?Any hx of heart disease?"*

<u>Alcohol</u> — *"Do you drink alcohol? How often do you drink alcohol?"*

Name / Age

PC - Empathy

SOCRATES———————————**Impact**

+ Delirium questions.

DDx **It's Me Sad**

↑

Other causes

↑

Psych Hx- **MOoAPS**

P A M H U G S F O S S

|

S A D

Delirium (Continued)

Infection, Trauma, Sx, Medication / LETO, Stroke, Alcohol, Drugs

I t 's Me S A D

<u>Drugs</u> — *"Have you done any recreational drugs? What have you used? How do you take it? Do you sniff or inject? Do you share needles?"*

Name / Age

PC - Empathy

SOCRATES—-------------------**Impact**

+ Delirium questions.

DDx **It's Me Sad**

↑

Other causes

↑

Psych Hx- MOoAPS

P A M   H U G S   F O S S

|

S A D

Suicide

SOCRATES + **SAD PERSONS** + MOoAPS Hx

SIGN POST *"Just to make sure there's nothing serious going on."*

Thyroid Anemia Medications Alcohol Drugs

T A Med A D

SIGN POST DDx: *"I'd like to ask you a few questions to rule out other causes."*

Thyroid — *"Have you had any thyroid issues in the past? Do you have any heat or cold tolerance?"*

Anemia — *"Do you find that you are paler than everyone else? Any hx of blood disorders? Do you bleed easily or bruise easily?"*

Medications — *"Are there any medications you take? Dosage/duration?"*

Alcohol — *"Do you drink alcohol? How often do you drink alcohol?"*

Drugs — *"Have you done any recreational drugs? What have you used? How do you take it? Do you sniff or inject? Do you share needles?"*

Name / Age

PC - Empathy

SOCRATES——------------------**Impact**

Confidentiality!

SAD PERSONS (≥ 5 - Hospitalize)

SIGN POST DDx T A Med AD

↑

Other causes

↑

Psych Hx- MOoAPS - C

'G CAT WAS SAD' -criteria for depression (≥ 5 for 2 weeks)

P A M   H U G S   F O S S

|

S A D

Insomnia

SOCRATES + CLARIFY - If it's difficulty falling asleep or waking up + Ask questions about sleep hygiene in the order of BEFORE, DURING, and AFTER.

BEFORE: *"Do you work night shifts? Is there a bedtime routine? When do you start to wind up? Do you eat before sleeping/heavy meals/late meals? Do you read in bed? Are you on your phone or looking at a screen?"*
DURING: *"How many hours do you sleep? Do you wake up during the night? How often? Do you snore? Did anyone ever notice you gasp for air while sleeping? Do you have any jerky movts? Any nightmares? Did you ever wake up screaming from your sleep? Did you ever walk in your sleep/perform tasks while sleeping?"*
AFTER: *"Do you feel unrefreshed or tired when waking up? Do you have any morning headaches? Did you ever notice hallucinations while drifting into sleep or drifting out of it? Did you ever collapse suddenly when excited or surprised?"*

Fatigue Anxiety Abuse insomnia Depression Sleep Disorder

F A A i D S

SIGN POST DDx: *"I'd like to ask you a few questions to rule out other causes."*

Name / Age

PC - Empathy

SOCRATES—-------------------**Impact**

For patients with sleep issues-

SIGN POST DDx F A A i D S

+ G CAT WAS SAD - criteria for depression (≥ 5 for 2 weeks) + MOoAPS Hx

P A M H U G S F O S S

S A D
caffeine

Fatigue

"Just to make sure there's nothing serious going on."

Anxiety, Abuse, Insomnia, Depression

A A I D

DDx: *"I'd like to ask you a few questions to rule out other causes."*

LMP, Meds, Anemia, RA, MM, PMR, Infection, Thyroid, SLE, Chronic

L Med A R M P I T S C

LMP — *"Are you pregnant by any chance? When was your LMP?"*

Medication — *"Are there any medications you take? Any changes to your prescription lately? Dosage/duration?"*

Anemia — *"Do you find that you are paler than everyone else? Any hx of blood disorders? Do you bleed easily or bruise easily?"*

Rheumatoid Arthritis (RA) — Morning stiffness lasts ↑ ½ hour. Symmetrical joint pain relieved by activity. Can ask about any nodules on fingers.

Name / Age

PC - Empathy

SOCRATES——------------------**Impact**

Clarify! Is it weakness during activity/lack of energy or feeling unrefreshed after sleep?

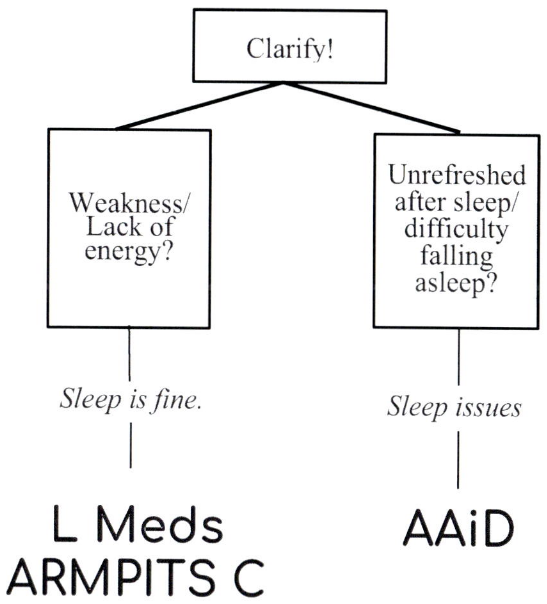

P A M H U G S F O S S

S A D

Fatigue (Continued)

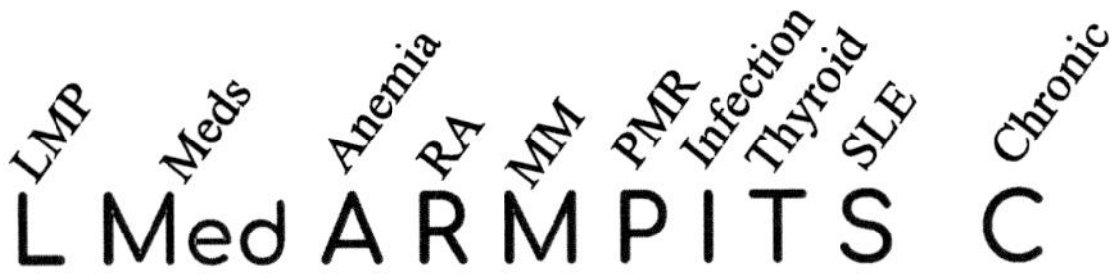

Multiple Myeloma (MM) — *"Have you experienced persistent bone pain, especially in your back, ribs and hips? Have you had frequent infections/ unexplained weight loss/ constipation or frequent urination?"*

Polymyalgia Rheumatica (PMR) — *"Do you have pain/ stiffness in both shoulders? Do you notice this more in the morning? Is this associated with fatigue/ fever/ weight loss? Do you have difficulty putting on a shirt?"*

Infection — *"Do you have a fever? Any hx of sick contacts? Any hx of travel?"*

Thyroid — *"Have you had any thyroid issues in the past? Do you have any heat or cold tolerance?"*

Systemic Lupus Erythematosus (SLE) — *"Have you noticed any rashes on your face or body? Have you experienced sensitivity to light? Have you noticed that your skin is paler than others? Have you had any oral ulcers? Any weakness/ fatigue/ fever?"* Also, check MSK Key -**MD SOAP PHEN**.

Chronic – (COPD, CLD, CKD) — *"Do you have any history of any chronic illness?"*

Name / Age

PC - Empathy

SOCRATES——————————**Impact**

Clarify! Is it weakness during activity/lack of energy or feeling unrefreshed after sleep?

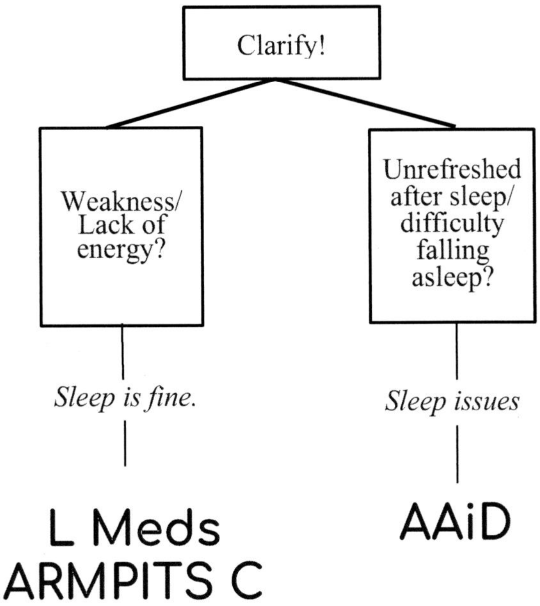

P A M   H U G S   F O S S

S A D

NOTES

Made in United States
Orlando, FL
04 November 2026

90214009R00148